Problem Solving in Cancer

Problem Solving
in Cancer
Immunotherapy

Edited by

Ruth E. Board, BSc, MBChB, PhD, FRCP
Consultant in Medical Oncology, Rosemere Cancer Centre, Royal Preston Hospital,
Lancashire Teaching Hospitals NHS Foundation Trust, Preston

Paul Nathan, BSc, BA, MBBS, PhD, FRCP
Consultant in Medical Oncology, Mount Vernon Cancer Centre, Northwood, Middlesex

Tom Newsom-Davis, BSc, MBBS, PhD, FRCP
Consultant in Medical Oncology, Chelsea and Westminster Hospital NHS Foundation
Trust, London

Sophie Papa, BA, MBBS, PhD, MRCP
Senior Lecturer in Immunotherapy-Oncology, King's College London, London; Honorary
Consultant in Medical Oncology, Guy's and St Thomas' NHS Foundation Trust, London

Peter Johnson, CBE, MD, FACP (UK), FRCP, FMedSci
Professor of Medical Oncology, Cancer Research UK Centre, University of Southampton,
Southampton

Published in association with the Association of Cancer Physicians

EBN HEALTH

OXFORD, UK

EBN Health
An imprint of Evidence-based Networks Ltd
Witney Business & Innovation Centre
Windrush House, Burford Road
Witney, Oxfordshire OX29 7DX, UK

Tel: +44 1865 522326
Email: info@ebnhealth.com

Web: www.ebnhealth.com

Distributed worldwide by:
Marston Book Services Ltd
160 Eastern Avenue
Milton Park
Abingdon
Oxon OX14 4SB, UK
Tel: +44 1235 465500
Fax: +44 1235 465555
Email: trade.orders@marston.co.uk

A catalogue record for this book is available from the British Library.

ISBN 13   978 0 99559 542 2

Series design by Pete Russell Typographic Design, Faringdon, Oxon, UK
Typeset by Thomson Digital, Noida, India
Printed by Latimer Trend and Company Ltd, Plymouth, UK

Contents

Contributors

Dr Helen Adderley, Specialist Registrar in Medical Oncology, Christie NHS Foundation Trust, Manchester

Dr Elizabeth Appleton, Registrar in Medical Oncology, Leeds Cancer Centre, St James's University Hospital, Leeds Teaching Hospitals NHS Trust, Leeds

Dr Lewis Au, Clinical Research Fellow, Royal Marsden NHS Foundation Trust, London

Dr Anna Beattie, Consultant in Cardiothoracic Radiology, Newcastle upon Tyne Hospitals NHS Foundation Trust, Newcastle upon Tyne

Dr Reuben Benjamin, Consultant in Haematology, King's College Hospital, London; Honorary Senior Lecturer, King's College London, London

Dr Alison May Berner, Academic Clinical Fellow and Specialty Trainee in Medical Oncology, Mount Vernon Cancer Centre, Northwood, Middlesex

Dr Ruth E. Board, Consultant in Medical Oncology, Rosemere Cancer Centre, Royal Preston Hospital, Lancashire Teaching Hospitals NHS Foundation Trust, Preston

Dr Rachel Broadbent, Specialist Registrar in Medical Oncology, Christie NHS Foundation Trust, Manchester

Dr Conor Broderick, Specialist Registrar in Dermatology, Addenbrooke's Hospital, Cambridge University Hospitals NHS Foundation Trust, Cambridge

Dr James Clark, Core Medical Trainee, Royal Marsden NHS Foundation Trust, London

Dr Claire M. Connell, Registrar in Medical Oncology, Addenbrooke's Hospital, Cambridge University Hospitals NHS Foundation Trust, Cambridge

Dr Pippa G. Corrie, Consultant and Associate Lecturer, Cambridge Cancer Trials Centre, Cambridge University Hospitals NHS Foundation Trust, Cambridge

Dr David Marc Davies, Postdoctoral Research Scientist, Research Oncology, King's College London, London

Dr Gary J. Doherty, Consultant in Medical Oncology, Addenbrooke's Hospital, Cambridge University Hospitals NHS Foundation Trust, Cambridge

Dr Joanne S. Evans, NIHR Academic Clinical Fellow in Medical Oncology, Chelsea and Westminster Hospital NHS Foundation Trust, London; NIHR Academic Clinical Fellow in Medical Oncology, Imperial College London, London

Professor John Gosney, Consultant in Thoracic Pathology, Royal Liverpool University Hospital, Royal Liverpool and Broadgreen University Hospitals NHS Trust, Liverpool; Professor of Thoracic Pathology, University of Liverpool, Liverpool

Dr Charlotte Graham, Clinical Research Fellow, King's College London, London

Dr Alastair Greystoke, Senior Lecturer and Honorary Consultant in Medical Oncology, Northern Centre for Cancer Care, Freeman Hospital, Newcastle upon Tyne Hospitals NHS Foundation Trust, Newcastle upon Tyne

Dr Avinash Gupta, Consultant in Medical Oncology, Christie NHS Foundation Trust, Manchester

Dr Alexander Haragan, Clinical Research Fellow in Pathology, Institute of Translational Medicine, Royal Liverpool and Broadgreen University Hospitals NHS Trust, Liverpool

Professor Robert Hawkins, Honorary Consultant in Medical Oncology, Cancer Research UK, Christie NHS Foundation Trust, Manchester

Dr Samuel L. Hill, Registrar in Medical Oncology, University Hospital Southampton NHS Foundation Trust, Southampton

Dr Satinder Jagdev, Consultant in Medical Oncology, Leeds Cancer Centre, St James's University Hospital, Leeds Teaching Hospitals NHS Trust, Leeds

Dr Adam P. Januszewski, Academic Clinical Fellow, Imperial College London; Academic Clinical Fellow, Royal Marsden NHS Foundation Trust, London

Professor Peter W.M. Johnson, Professor of Medical Oncology, Cancer Research UK Centre, University of Southampton, Southampton

Dr Rebecca Johnson, Core Medical Trainee, Oxford Cancer and Haematology Centre, Oxford University Hospitals NHS Foundation Trust, Oxford

Professor Rob J. Jones, Honorary Consultant in Medical Oncology, Beatson West of Scotland Cancer Centre, Glasgow; Professor of Clinical Cancer Research, University of Glasgow, Glasgow

Dr Ioannis Karydis, Honorary Consultant in Medical Oncology, University Hospital Southampton NHS Trust, Southampton; Associate Professor in Oncology, University of Southampton, Southampton

Dr Beth Lambourne, Registrar in Medical Oncology, Northern Centre for Cancer Care, Freeman Hospital, Newcastle upon Tyne Hospitals NHS Foundation Trust, Newcastle upon Tyne

Dr James Larkin, Consultant in Medical Oncology, Royal Marsden NHS Foundation Trust, London

Dr Maria Marples, Consultant in Medical Oncology, Leeds Cancer Centre, St James's University Hospital, Leeds Teaching Hospitals NHS Trust, Leeds

Dr Maria Martinez, Registrar in Medical Oncology, Beatson West of Scotland Cancer Centre, Glasgow

Professor Alan Melcher, Professor of Translational Immunotherapy, Institute of Cancer Research, London

Dr Romaana Mir, Research Fellow in Melanoma, Mount Vernon Cancer Centre, Northwood, Middlesex

Dr Dan R. Muller, Fellow in Immune Oncology, University Hospital Southampton NHS Foundation Trust, Southampton

Dr Paul D. Nathan, Consultant in Medical Oncology, Mount Vernon Cancer Centre, Northwood, Middlesex

Dr Tom Newsom-Davis, Consultant in Medical Oncology, Chelsea and Westminster Hospital NHS Foundation Trust, London

Dr Anna Olsson-Brown, Registrar in Medical Oncology, Clatterbridge Cancer Centre NHS Foundation Trust, Birkenhead; Clinical Research Fellow, University of Liverpool, Liverpool

Professor Christian Ottensmeier, Professor of Experimental Cancer Medicine, NIHR and Cancer Research UK Experimental Cancer Medicine Centre, Southampton University Hospitals NHS Foundation Trust, Southampton

Dr Sophie Papa, Senior Lecturer in Immunotherapy-Oncology, King's College London, London; Honorary Consultant in Medical Oncology, Guy's and St Thomas' NHS Foundation Trust, London

Dr Alec Paschalis, Specialty Registrar in Medical Oncology, University Hospital Southampton NHS Foundation Trust, Southampton

Dr Miranda Payne, Consultant in Medical Oncology, Oxford Cancer and Haematology Centre, Oxford University Hospitals NHS Foundation Trust, Oxford

Dr Magnus Pedersen, PhD Student, Center for Cancer Immune Therapy, Departments of Hematology and Oncology, Herlev and Gentofte Hospital, Herlev, Denmark

Dr Benjamin Pickwell-Smith, Specialist Registrar in Medical Oncology, Christie NHS Foundation Trust, Manchester

Dr Manon Pillai, Specialist Registrar in Medical Oncology, Christie NHS Foundation Trust, Manchester

Dr Sanjay Popat, Consultant in Medical Oncology, Royal Marsden NHS Foundation Trust, London

Dr Christy Ralph, Consultant in Medical Oncology, Leeds Cancer Centre, St James's University Hospital, Leeds Teaching Hospitals NHS Trust, Leeds

Dr John Reicher, Specialty Registrar in Clinical Radiology, Freeman Hospital, Newcastle upon Tyne Hospitals NHS Foundation Trust, Newcastle upon Tyne

Dr Marcus Remer, Specialty Registrar in Medical Oncology, University Hospital Southampton NHS Foundation Trust, Southampton

Dr Joseph Sacco, Honorary Consultant in Medical Oncology, Clatterbridge Cancer Centre, NHS Foundation Trust, Birkenhead; Clinical Senior Lecturer, University of Liverpool, Liverpool

Dr Zena Salih, Specialist Registrar in Medical Oncology, Christie NHS Foundation Trust, Manchester

Dr Amit Samani, Academic Clinical Fellow in Medical Oncology, King's College London, London

Dr Adel Samson, Honorary Consultant in Medical Oncology, Leeds Cancer Centre, St James's University Hospital, Leeds Teaching Hospitals NHS Trust, Leeds; Academic Fellow, University of Leeds, Leeds

Professor Peter Selby, Professor of Cancer Medicine, Leeds Cancer Centre, St James's University Hospital, Leeds Teaching Hospitals NHS Trust, Leeds; Associate Dean, Leeds Institute of Cancer and Pathology, University of Leeds, Leeds

Dr Anand Sharma, Consultant in Medical Oncology, Mount Vernon Cancer Centre, Northwood, Middlesex

Dr Heather M. Shaw, Consultant in Medical Oncology, University College London Hospitals NHS Foundation Trust, London

Dr Beth Shepherd, Consultant Oncological Radiologist, Southampton General Hospital, University Hospital Southampton NHS Foundation Trust, Southampton

Dr Alfred C.P. So, Foundation Year 1 Doctor, Queen's Hospital, Barking, Havering and Redbridge University Hospitals NHS Trust, Romford, Essex

Dr Ally Speight, Consultant in Gastroenterology, Newcastle upon Tyne Hospitals NHS Foundation Trust, Newcastle upon Tyne

Dr Pavlina Spiliopoulou, Registrar in Medical Oncology, Beatson West of Scotland Cancer Centre, Glasgow

Dr Rosalind Stewart, Consultant in Ophthalmology, Leeds Centre for Ophthalmology, St James's University Hospital, Leeds Teaching Hospitals NHS Trust, Leeds

Dr Claire Storey, Specialist Trainee in Respiratory Medicine, Freeman Hospital, Newcastle upon Tyne Hospitals NHS Foundation Trust, Newcastle upon Tyne

Dr Fiona Thistlethwaite, Consultant in Medical Oncology, Christie NHS Foundation Trust, Manchester; Honorary Senior Lecturer, University of Manchester, Manchester

Dr Jennifer Thomas, Clinical Research Fellow, Royal Marsden NHS Foundation Trust, London

Dr Balaji Venugopal, Consultant in Medical Oncology, Beatson West of Scotland Cancer Centre, Glasgow; Honorary Clinical Senior Lecturer, University of Glasgow, Glasgow

Dr Andrew Viggars, Specialty Registrar in Medical Oncology, Huddersfield Royal Infirmary, Calderdale and Huddersfield NHS Foundation Trust, Huddersfield

Professor Richard Vile, Professor of Immunology, Mayo Clinic, Rochester, MN, USA

Dr Marc Wallace, Consultant in Dermatology, Addenbrooke's Hospital, Cambridge University Hospitals NHS Foundation Trust, Cambridge

Professor Andrew M. Wardley, Professor in Breast Medical Oncology, Manchester Academic Health Science Centre, Manchester; Consultant in Medical Oncology, Christie NHS Foundation Trust, Manchester; Honorary Professor, University of Manchester, Manchester

Dr Sarah J. Welsh, Consultant in Medical Oncology, Cambridge University Hospitals NHS Foundation Trust, Cambridge

Dr Matthew Wheater, Consultant in Medical Oncology, University Hospital Southampton NHS Foundation Trust, Southampton

Dr Sunnya Zarif, Registrar in Medical Oncology, University Hospital Southampton NHS Foundation Trust, Southampton

Preface

In recent years there has been a paradigm shift in the treatment of cancer as immunotherapy drugs have taken centre stage. The success of harnessing a patient's own immune system has led to an unprecedented expansion of treatment options for both solid and haematological malignancies. Immune checkpoint inhibitors in particular have been shown to improve outcomes in patients with a range of tumours and are in routine first line use in a number of malignancies. The development of genetically modified T cell therapy has demonstrated real advances in the treatment of haematological malignancies and, although in its infancy in the treatment of solid tumours, early successes have shown promising results.

Much excitement has centred around the observation of durable, long-term response to immunotherapy. With longer-term follow-up the suggestion of cancer cure in some patients has become a real possibility. There remain, however, challenges in the introduction of immunotherapies into standard clinical practice. While many immunotherapy drugs have been shown to be better tolerated than cytotoxic chemotherapies or targeted agents, the side effects experienced are very different from those traditionally observed with anticancer agents. Education of oncology teams and the wider medical community is paramount in ensuring early detection and correct management of side effects. Discovery of robust biomarkers to identify patients most likely to benefit from immunotherapies and those in whom side effects may occur remains elusive. The optimism created by the arrival of immunotherapy is real and justified but has also created practical problems, as patients may remain on treatment and follow-up for many years. This is a gratifying situation to be in, but one which requires increased resources for treatment units, and places an increased financial burden on healthcare systems.

This most recent book in the Association of Cancer Physicians' prize-winning *Problem Solving* series seeks to provide the reader with a review of the most up-to-date issues and challenges in immunotherapy treatments. Twelve chapters, written by leading authorities in the field, give an overview of the development of immunotherapy at a molecular, clinical and patient-centred level. Twenty-three individual case histories are then used to illustrate how immunotherapy has been successful across a range of tumour types, highlighting evidence-based practice and illustrating how immune-related side effects are managed in the clinic.

This is a fast-moving area of cancer treatment and we have captured the most recent findings and highlighted future developments to help healthcare professionals understand this evolving field. Our purpose has been to provide a highly readable text that is accessible and understandable for anyone interested in this exciting area of novel cancer treatment.

Ruth Board, Paul Nathan, Tom Newsom-Davis, Sophie Papa and Peter Johnson, Editors
David Cunningham, Chairman, Association of Cancer Physicians
Peter Selby, President, Association of Cancer Physicians

Acknowledgements

Editors

The editors and authors are grateful to all the patients who have inspired them to prepare this book and work together to improve patient care.

The editors, authors and publisher are most grateful to the Executive Committee of the Association of Cancer Physicians for their support and advice during development of the book.

We are grateful to Duncan Enright and Beverley Martin at EBN Health for their expert work, support, goodwill and interest in our purpose in preparing the book, and Nicole Goldman, who coordinated and oversaw the book's preparation and organization.

Dr Board would like to acknowledge the support of the University of Manchester and Lancashire Teaching Hospitals NHS Foundation Trust. Dr Nathan would like to acknowledge the support of his colleagues at Mount Vernon Cancer Centre. Dr Newsom-Davis would like to acknowledge the support of Chelsea and Westminster Hospital NHS Foundation Trust. Dr Papa would like to acknowledge the support of Guy's and St Thomas' NHS Foundation Trust, King's College London, King's Health Partners' Cancer Research UK Centre and the Medical Research Council. Professor Johnson would like to acknowledge the support of Cancer Research UK, the University of Southampton and University Hospital Southampton NHS Foundation Trust.

Ruth Board, Paul Nathan, Tom Newsom-Davis, Sophie Papa and Peter Johnson

Association of Cancer Physicians

The *Problem Solving* series of cancer-related books is developed and prepared by the Association of Cancer Physicians, often in partnership with one or more other specialist medical organizations. As the representative body for medical oncologists in the UK, the Association of Cancer Physicians has a broad set of aims, including education for its own members and for non-members, including interested clinicians, healthcare professionals and the public. The *Problem Solving* series is a planned sequence of publications that derive from a programme of annual scientific workshops initiated in 2014 with 'Problem Solving in Acute Oncology' followed by 'Problem Solving in Older Cancer Patients', 'Problem Solving Through Precision Oncology', 'Problem Solving in Patient-Centred and Integrated Cancer Care' and, most recently, 'Problem Solving in Immunotherapy'.

The publications involve considerable work from members and other contributors; this work is done without remuneration, as an educational service. The books have been well received and we are delighted with their standard. *Problem Solving in Older Cancer Patients* and *Problem Solving Through Precision Oncology* were awarded the BMA prize for best oncology book of the year in 2016 and 2017, respectively.

The Association of Cancer Physicians wishes to thank all the contributors to this and previous publications and those yet to come.

David Cunningham, Chairman, Association of Cancer Physicians
Peter Selby, President, Association of Cancer Physicians

Abbreviations

ACT	Adoptive T cell therapy	ECOG	Eastern Cooperative Oncology Group
ACTH	Adrenocorticotropic hormone		
ADC	Antibody–drug conjugate	EGF	Epidermal growth factor
AJCC	American Joint Committee on Cancer	ER	Oestrogen receptor
		ERK	Extracellular signal-regulated kinase
AKI	Acute kidney injury	ESMO	European Society for Medical Oncology
ALL	Acute lymphoblastic leukaemia		
ALT	Alanine aminotransferase	FDA	Food and Drug Administration
AML	Acute myeloid leukaemia	FDG	Fluorodeoxyglucose
APC	Antigen-presenting cell	FOXP3	Forkhead box P3
APOBEC	Apolipoprotein B mRNA-editing enzyme, catalytic polypeptide-like	GCSF	Granulocyte colony-stimulating factor
AST	Aspartate aminotransferase	GITR	Glucocorticoid-induced tumour necrosis factor receptor-related protein
B-ALL	B cell acute lymphoblastic leukaemia		
BCG	*Bacillus* Calmette–Guérin	GM-CSF	Granulocyte macrophage colony-stimulating factor
BCMA	B cell membrane antigen		
B-NHL	B cell non-Hodgkin lymphoma	gp	Glycoprotein
BNP	Brain natriuretic peptide	HAVCR2	Hepatitis A virus cellular receptor 2
BRAF	Serine/threonine-protein kinase B-Raf	HD IL-2	High-dose interleukin-2
		HER2	Human epidermal growth factor receptor 2
CAR	Chimeric antigen receptor		
CD	Cluster of differentiation	HLA	Human leucocyte antigen
CEA	Carcinoembryonic antigen	HMGB1	High mobility group box 1
CEACAM1	Carcinoembryonic antigen-related cell adhesion molecule 1	HPV	Human papilloma virus
		HSV-1	Herpes simplex virus type 1
CIS	Cytokine-inducible SH2-containing protein	ICP	Infected cell protein
		ICPI	Immune checkpoint inhibitor
CLL	Chronic lymphocytic leukaemia	IDO	Indoleamine 2,3-dioxygenase
CM	Cutaneous melanoma	IFN	Interferon
CMR	Cardiac magnetic resonance	IL	Interleukin
CMV	Cytomegalovirus	IL-13Rα2	Interleukin-13 receptor subunit α2
COP	Cryptogenic organizing pneumonia	IL-6R	Interleukin-6 receptor
CRP	C-reactive protein	irAE	Immune-related adverse event
CRS	Cytokine release syndrome	iRECIST	Immune-based Response Evaluation Criteria in Solid Tumors
CTCAE	Common Terminology Criteria for Adverse Events		
		JAK-STAT	Janus kinase–signal transducers and activators of transcription
CTLA-4	Cytotoxic T lymphocyte-associated protein 4		
		LAG	Lymphocyte-activation gene protein
DLBCL	Diffuse large B cell lymphoma	LDH	Lactate dehydrogenase

MAGE	Melanoma-associated antigen	PJP	*Pneumocystis jirovecii* pneumonia
MAGE-A3	Melanoma-associated antigen 3	PR	Progesterone receptor
MAPK	Mitogen-activated protein kinase	RCC	Renal cell carcinoma
MART-1	Melanoma antigen recognized by T cells 1	RCT	Randomized controlled trial
		RECIST	Response Evaluation Criteria in Solid Tumors
MEK	Mitogen-activated protein kinase kinase		
		RGMb	Repulsive guidance molecule B
MHC	Major histocompatibility complex	SCAD	Segmental colitis associated with diverticulosis
MMM	Mucosal malignant melanoma		
MRCP	Magnetic resonance cholangiopancreatography	scFv	Single-chain variable fragment
		SHP	Src homology region 2-containing protein tyrosine phosphatase
MVAC	Methotrexate, vinblastine, doxorubicin, cisplatin		
		SNP	Single nucleotide polymorphism
NFAT	Nuclear factor of activated T cells	TAA	Tumour-associated antigen
NFκB	Nuclear factor κB	TCR	T cell receptor
NHL	Non-Hodgkin lymphoma	TGF	Transforming growth factor
NK	Natural killer	TIGIT	T cell immunoreceptor with immunoglobulin and ITIM domains
NSCLC	Non-small-cell lung carcinoma		
OS	Overall survival		
OX40	Tumour necrosis factor receptor superfamily, member 4	TIL	Tumour-infiltrating lymphocyte
		TIM	T cell immunoglobulin and mucin domain
PBMC	Peripheral blood mononuclear cell		
PD-1	Programmed cell death protein 1	TKI	Tyrosine kinase inhibitor
PD-L1	Programmed death-ligand 1	TNF	Tumour necrosis factor
PD-L2	Programmed death-ligand 2	TSA	Tumour-specific antigen
PFS	Progression-free survival	T-VEC	Talimogene laherparepvec
PFU	Plaque-forming unit	ULN	Upper limit of normal
PI3K	Phosphoinositide 3-kinase	VEGF	Vascular endothelial growth factor

The editors would like to dedicate this book to
Professor Peter Selby CBE.

As president of the Association of Cancer Physicians it has been
Peter's vision to develop a series of workshops and educational books
based on real life case studies to provide medical oncology trainees and
the wider medical community with a superb, award-winning resource.

01 Immunotherapy: Past, Present and Future

Samuel L. Hill, Peter W.M. Johnson

Past

The intuitive appeal of eliciting an effective immune response against cancers has long been recognized but, until quite recently, rarely fulfilled. At the end of the 19th century, William Coley, a New York sarcoma surgeon, noted some tumour regressions in cancer patients infected with streptococci, by provoking an immune response.[1] But such responses proved hard to replicate and his treatments quickly fell out of favour. The idea, however, remained potent. Occasional instances of spontaneous tumour regression[2,3] or prolonged dormancy suggested some form of 'host restraint', and a number of clinical successes kept the field of immunotherapy alive, despite the many failed attempts at treatment.

As the science of immunology developed, together with an emerging understanding of the innate and adaptive immune system, so interest in its function in modulating tumours was rekindled. The use of intravesical *Bacillus* Calmette–Guérin (BCG) to stimulate regression of superficial bladder cancers was the first true immunotherapy to be adopted, in the 1960s. The mechanism of spontaneous regression was investigated and, with a viral aetiology for cancer suspected, antibodies were thought to play a key role, as were newly discovered cytokines and other signalling peptides.[2]

The invention of hybridoma technology in 1975[4] overcame previous difficulties in making large quantities of specific immunoglobulin, allowing antibodies directly targeting tumour antigens to be tested for the first time. The results were initially disappointing, owing to the short half-life and poor recruitment of human immune effector mechanisms by murine antibodies; however, with the development of molecules including human constant regions more successes were seen, such as the targeting of clusters of differentiation (CD) 52 antigens on lymphoma by the Campath-1H antibody.[5]

Despite theoretical reservations about the depletion of normal B cells and poor effector capacity in patients with advanced lymphoma, rituximab proved an effective treatment for B cell malignancies, in 1997 becoming the first monoclonal antibody to be licensed for use in humans. This chimeric monoclonal antibody, targeting CD20, has several mechanisms of action once attached to the target cell, activating antibody-dependent cytotoxicity and complement-dependent cytotoxicity, as well as driving apoptosis.[6] Its impact in improving survival from B cell lymphomas has been so marked that it has been classified by the WHO as an essential medicine.[7,8] Subsequently, an ever-increasing number of monoclonal antibodies targeting cancer cells themselves have been licensed. They either evoke effector mechanisms, in a similar manner to that of rituximab, or act by inhibiting aspecific stimulatory pathways, such as the use of trastuzumab to block activation of the epidermal growth factor (EGF) pathway in human epidermal growth factor receptor 2 (HER2)-positive breast cancer.[9]

In the 1990s, through the work of groups at the Ludwig Institute for Cancer Research, in Brussels, and others, it became apparent that malignant cells do evoke responses by CD8-positive cytotoxic T cells and CD4-positive T helper cells through presentation of self peptides via major histocompatibility complex (MHC) class I and class II molecules, respectively. These peptides are derived from proteins of low or tissue-restricted expression in the adult, such as the melanoma-associated antigen (MAGE) family of proteins found only on testicular tissue and cancers.[10] A number of such peptides were identified by expression cloning from T cells in tumour-bearing individuals, leading to the development of potential vaccine strategies using proteins, peptides or nucleic acids. Molecules such as the melanocyte-restricted gp100 antigen and melanoma antigen recognized by T cells 1 (MART-1) were tested clinically, but to modest effect and with low response rates, leading many to turn away from this approach.[11]

One vaccine strategy that has been slightly more effective is the use of autologous peripheral blood mononuclear cells (PBMCs), loaded with tumour cell line protein preparations or cancer antigens to enrich and activate professional antigen-presenting cells (APCs). This has been approved in the form of the sipuleucel-T vaccine, in which PBMCs are activated with prostatic acid phosphatase fused to recombinant granulocyte macrophage colony-stimulating factor (GM-CSF), which has shown a small survival advantage when given to men with metastatic prostate cancer.[12]

As the search for the cause of spontaneous tumour regressions continued, molecules that could modulate tumours *in vivo* were discovered, notably interleukin (IL)-2 and interferon (IFN)-α. The systemic or topical administration of cytokines was investigated in large-scale clinical trials in the 1980s, with mixed results. IFN-α was shown to have multiple effector functions, including immunoregulatory, antiproliferative, differentiation-inducing, apoptotic and antiangiogenic properties, across multiple malignancies. Toxicities with such treatments were substantial and response rates were low in advanced disease. In phase I and II trials in metastatic melanoma, objective response rates were reported to be between 10% and 20%, with some appearing durable.[13] In 1986, the US Food and Drug Administration approved IFN-α2 for the treatment of hairy cell leukaemia and subsequently in 1995 as adjuvant treatment for stage IIB/III melanoma. IL-2 was the second exogenous cytokine approved for use in treatment of solid tumours, including melanoma and renal cell carcinoma (RCC).[14]

With improved understanding of the human T cell response to cancer, alternative approaches to cytotoxic T lymphocyte activation were explored. The feedback control mechanisms for such responses were recognized as potential targets for antibody blockade and the first immune checkpoint inhibitors (ICPIs) were developed. The cytotoxic T lymphocyte-associated protein 4 (CTLA-4)-specific antibody ipilimumab was tested, with striking responses in some individuals with widespread melanoma,[15] leading to its licensing in 2011 and heralding the start of the modern era of cancer immunotherapy (Figure 1.1).

Present

It is apparent that despite many tumours eliciting a cytotoxic T cell response they remain able to avoid detection and destruction as they develop and evolve in the host. Such immune evasion may occur either through selective immune tolerance or by resistance to immune targeting. Immune editing reflects the evolution of cancers in response to their microenvironment, with genomic alterations, activation of numerous cytokines or chemokines, and expression of other molecules to produce tolerance by the immune system. The complex interplay that

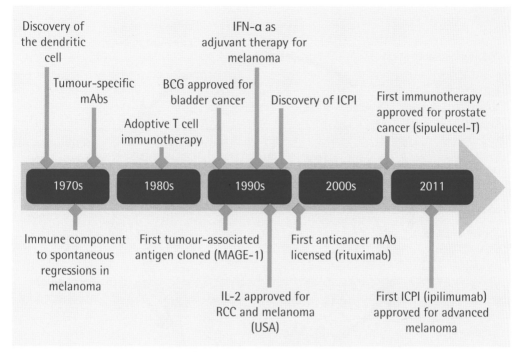

Figure 1.1 Key events in the development of immunotherapy (adapted from Kirkwood *et al.*[2]). mAb, monoclonal antibody.

allows either tolerance or immune destruction of a cancer has been described by Chen and Mellman[16] as a cancer immunity cycle, numerous points on which are now being targeted for therapy (Figure 1.2).

Following the success of ipilimumab targeting CTLA-4, antibodies blocking programmed cell death protein 1 (PD-1) and its ligand programmed death-ligand 1 (PD-L1) have been developed and also demonstrate impressive results in some tumour types. The combination of ipilimumab with nivolumab, an anti-PD-1 antibody, has shown a significant improvement in the response rate for patients treated for metastatic melanoma, and most importantly an increase in survival, recently recorded as a 3 year survival of 58% in previously untreated advanced disease.[17]

Such results in cancers with previously poor outcomes have resulted in ICPIs being tested in almost all types of malignancy, alone, in combination, or with other treatment modalities, conventional or experimental. As of September 2017 there were more than 1500 clinical trials in progress targeting the PD-1/PD-L1 pathway.[18] ICPIs are now licensed for use in a number of indications, including melanoma, non-small-cell lung carcinoma, malignancies of the urinary tract, head and neck cancers, and Hodgkin's lymphoma. It has become clear that particular malignancies respond better than others to ICPI treatment, especially those with a high degree of genomic damage and high mutational burden. For example, tumours with microsatellite instability and those with deficiency in DNA mismatch repair, either through germline or somatic mutations, have shown higher response rates.[19] This has resulted in approval of the anti-PD-1 antibody pembrolizumab in the treatment of any cancer displaying this phenotype, irrespective of the site of

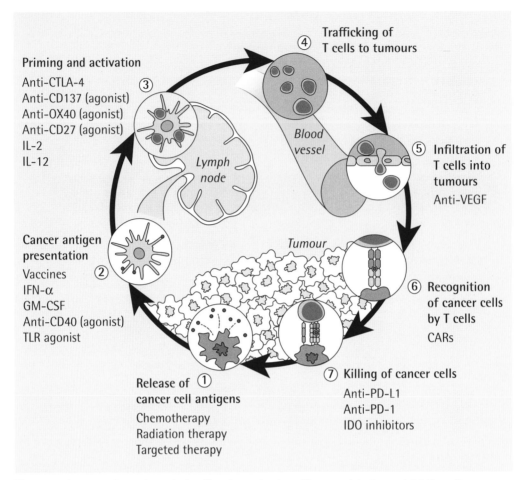

Figure 1.2 The cancer immunity cycle detailing the mechanism of immune detection and deletion of tumours. Highlighted are therapies currently in clinical use as well as in clinical and preclinical development (adapted from Chen and Mellman[16]). IDO, indoleamine 2,3-dioxygenase; TLR, toll-like receptor; VEGF, vascular endothelial growth factor.

origin. This is the first time an anticancer treatment has been approved for widespread use based on molecular phenotype alone.

The successful use of monoclonal antibodies targeting cancer cells and the refinement of the chemistry of molecular linkers have given rise to a new generation of antibody–drug conjugate (ADC) treatments. The construct ado-trastuzumab emtansine, combining trastuzumab with a microtubule inhibitor, has proven to be effective in the treatment of HER2 receptor-positive breast cancer.[20] Brentuximab vedotin, an anti-CD30 antibody linked to an anti-tubulin agent, has proven highly active in Hodgkin's lymphoma.[21] Clinical trials investigating further ADCs for targeted delivery of potent cytotoxics and radionuclides are ongoing.

The promise of harvesting and enhancing a patient's own immune effectors has been understood since the 1970s, when the discovery of the stimulatory effects of IL-2 were noted and preclinical trials demonstrated the effects of adoptively transferred lymphocytes. Tumour regressions were seen in selected patients whose melanomas were treated using expanded autologous tumour-infiltrating lymphocytes (TILs), which produced even greater improvements when treatment was preceded by lymphodepleting chemotherapy.[22] In an attempt to broaden the targets for adoptive cell therapy, the use of chimeric antigen receptors (CARs) was developed in the late 1980s. By linking the variable regions of antibody heavy and light chains to T cell receptor (TCR) signalling molecules such as CD3ζ, in combination with co-stimulatory domains such CD28 or 4–1BB, it was possible to direct cytotoxic T lymphocytes to non-MHC-restricted targets. This has been most successful in targeting the B cell antigen CD19, present on the surface of acute lymphoblastic leukaemia (ALL) and lymphomas.

Clinical studies of CAR T cell therapy have shown that it is a powerful treatment. Not only were response rates significant in patients with chemorefractory B cell malignancies, the side effects were also considerable, with symptoms associated with a profound cytokine release syndrome including significant neurotoxicity.[23] Recent trials have paved the way to the licensing of commercial T cell therapy targeting CD19 in the form of axicabtagene ciloleucel in diffuse large B cell lymphoma,[24] and tisagenlecleucel for ALL,[25] both in the relapsed or refractory setting.

Future

As we gain greater mechanistic understanding of the immune system and its complex interaction with cancers, we are making progress towards ever more targeted and specific treatments. The ability to overcome T cell anergy using ICPIs targeting CTLA-4 and PD-1/PD-L1 has changed the landscape of cancer treatment but is still a relatively non-specific approach which depends on a degree of pre-existing recognition of the tumour by T cells. These targets represent just two of a host of known immunomodulatory pathways that may yield other promising targets in the tumour microenvironment, in particular stimulatory targets capable of amplifying responses such as 4–1BB, CD27 and tumour necrosis factor receptor superfamily, member 4 (OX40), and other inhibitory molecules such as T cell immunoglobulin and mucin domain 3 (TIM-3), lymphocyte-activation gene (LAG)-3 protein and glucocorticoid-induced tumour necrosis factor receptor-related protein (GITR).[26] The latter have a role in inhibiting effector T cells and are also upregulated on regulatory T cells, depletion of which may be an alternative mechanism for amplifying anti-tumour responses.

Cancer vaccines, largely forgotten during the recent focus on ICPIs, may provide a means to drive more antigen-specific responses. Vaccines made from nucleic acid, peptides, proteins and dendritic cells are again under investigation across a range of tumour types.[27] Vaccine strategies have previously exploited a variety of tumour-associated antigens that are overexpressed in tumours but that may also be present at low levels in healthy tissues. This may lead to normal tissue targeting as well as T cell tolerance. The ability to rapidly sequence the whole genome of tumour cells and predict the peptides that will be effectively processed and presented has led to the development of strategies to target individual tumour-specific neoepitopes, generated by somatic mutations producing novel peptides that may be recognized by cytotoxic T cells.[28,29]

Crucial to the development of any cancer treatment is the ability to determine which patients are likely to gain most benefit from therapy and which are most likely to develop toxicities. The development of predictive biomarkers for immunotherapy is an active area of research. Tumour expression of PD-L1 is embedded in clinical practice but is not without its challenges, and future work will be essential to determine tumour- and blood-based biomarkers to guide treatment.

Critical to techniques characterizing the tumour mutanome is the need for powerful immunoinformatics. The ability to analyse large amounts of data from sources such as next generation sequencing, protein expression and TCR sequencing will lead to greater understanding of tumour biology and its interaction with its microenvironment. It is hoped this will lead to greater understanding of how some cancers remain devoid of infiltration by immune effector cells while others, even with high levels of TILs, remain unresponsive to immunotherapies.

As the complex interplay between a tumour and its surrounding tissues is dissected, we expect it will become increasingly possible to interfere and influence this process therapeutically. It is likely that this will include more than one technique in combination, to augment the response; the timing of these will be crucial, whether through inhibition of regulatory T cells, targeting antigens with novel ADCs or CAR T cells, or stimulation through peptide or APC vaccines. The next few years will see a massive expansion of combination immunotherapy approaches as well as combinations of immunotherapy with traditional cytotoxic and radiotherapy treatments.

References

1 McCarthy EF. The toxins of William B. Coley and the treatment of bone and soft-tissue sarcomas. *Iowa Orthop J* 2006; 26: 154–8.

2 Kirkwood JM, Butterfield LH, Tarhini AA, Zarour H. Immunotherapy of cancer in 2012. *CA Cancer J Clin* 2012; 62: 309–35.

3 Nathanson L. Spontaneous regression of malignant melanoma: a review of the literature on incidence, clinical features, and possible mechanisms. *Natl Cancer Inst Monogr* 1976; 44: 67–76.

4 Köhler G, Milstein C. Continuous cultures of fused cells secreting antibody of predefined specificity. *Nature* 1975; 256: 495–7.

5 Hale G, Dyer MJ, Clark MR, *et al.* Remission induction in non-Hodgkin lymphoma with reshaped human monoclonal antibody CAMPATH-1H. *Lancet* 1988; 2: 1394–9.

6 Lim SH, Beers SA, French RR, *et al.* Anti-CD20 monoclonal antibodies: historical and future perspectives. *Haematologica* 2010; 95: 135–43.

7 Coiffier B, Lepage E, Brière J, *et al.* CHOP chemotherapy plus rituximab compared with CHOP alone in elderly patients with diffuse large B-cell lymphoma. *N Engl J Med* 2002; 346: 235–42.

8 World Health Organization (2017). *WHO model lists of essential medicines. 20th list.* Available from: www.who.int/medicines/publications/essentialmedicines/20th_EML2017_FINAL_amendedAug2017.pdf?ua=1 (accessed 12 July 2018).

9 Hudis CA. Trastuzumab – mechanism of action and use in clinical practice. *N Engl J Med* 2007; 357: 39–51.

10 Boon T, Cerottini JC, Van den Eynde B, *et al.* Tumor antigens recognized by T lymphocytes. *Annu Rev Immunol* 1994; 12: 337–65.

11 Rosenberg SA, Yang JC, Restifo NP. Cancer immunotherapy: moving beyond current vaccines. *Nature Med* 2004; 10: 909–15.

12 Kantoff PW, Higano CS, Shore ND, *et al.* Sipuleucel-T immunotherapy for castration-resistant prostate cancer. *N Engl J Med* 2010; 363: 411–22.

13 Garbe C, Eigentler TK, Keilholz U, *et al.* Systematic review of medical treatment in melanoma: current status and future prospects. *Oncologist* 2011; 16: 5–24.

14 Rosenberg SA, Yang JC, Topalian SL, *et al*. Treatment of 283 consecutive patients with metastatic melanoma or renal cell cancer using high-dose bolus interleukin 2. *JAMA* 1994; 271: 907–13.

15 Hodi FS, O'Day SJ, McDermott DF, *et al*. Improved survival with ipilimumab in patients with metastatic melanoma. *N Engl J Med* 2010; 363: 711–23.

16 Chen DS, Mellman I. Oncology meets immunology: the cancer-immunity cycle. *Immunity* 2013; 39: 1–10.

17 Wolchok JD, Chiarion-Sileni V, González R, *et al*. Overall survival with combined nivolumab and ipilimumab in advanced melanoma. *N Engl J Med* 2017; 377: 1345–56.

18 Tang J, Shalabi A, Hubbard-Lucey VM. Comprehensive analysis of the clinical immuno-oncology landscape. *Ann Oncol* 2017; 29: 84–91.

19 Le DT, Uram JN, Wang H, *et al*. PD-1 blockade in tumors with mismatch-repair deficiency. *N Engl J Med* 2015; 372: 2509–20.

20 Lambert JM, Morris CQ. Antibody–drug conjugates (ADCs) for personalized treatment of solid tumors: a review. *Adv Ther* 2017; 34: 1015–35.

21 Connors JM, Jurczak W, Straus DJ, *et al*. Brentuximab vedotin with chemotherapy for stage III or IV Hodgkin's lymphoma. *N Engl J Med* 2018; 378: 331–44.

22 Rosenberg SA, Restifo NP. Adoptive cell transfer as personalized immunotherapy for human cancer. *Science* 2015; 348: 62–8.

23 Grupp SA, Kalos M, Barrett D, *et al*. Chimeric antigen receptor-modified T cells for acute lymphoid leukemia. *N Engl J Med* 2013; 368: 1509–18.

24 Neelapu SS, Locke FL, Bartlett NL, *et al*. Axicabtagene ciloleucel CAR T-cell therapy in refractory large B-cell lymphoma. *N Engl J Med* 2017; 377: 2531–44.

25 Maude SL, Laetsch TW, Buechner J, *et al*. Tisagenlecleucel in children and young adults with B-cell lymphoblastic leukemia. *N Engl J Med* 2018; 378: 439–48.

26 Melero I, Hervas-Stubbs S, Glennie M, *et al*. Immunostimulatory monoclonal antibodies for cancer therapy. *Nature Rev Cancer* 2007; 7: 95–106.

27 Marin-Acevedo JA, Soyano AE, Dholaria B, *et al*. Cancer immunotherapy beyond immune checkpoint inhibitors. *J Hematol Oncol* 2018; 11: 8.

28 Ott PA, Hu Z, Keskin DB, *et al*. An immunogenic personal neoantigen vaccine for patients with melanoma. *Nature* 2017; 547: 217–21.

29 Sahin U, Derhovanessian E, Miller M, *et al*. Personalized RNA mutanome vaccines mobilize poly-specific therapeutic immunity against cancer. *Nature* 2017; 547: 222–6.

02 Beyond Exhausted: Tumour Immune Checkpoints and Their Therapeutic Targets

Joanne S. Evans, Tom Newsom-Davis

Background

Immune checkpoint inhibitors (ICPIs) have transformed the treatment of a range of cancers, including melanoma, non-small-cell lung carcinoma and transitional cell carcinoma. Understanding their mechanism of action at a molecular level allows us to better appreciate their clinical behaviour and to identify the next generation of immunotherapy agents.

The primary mediator of the immune response is the activated T cell, which expresses a multitude of different co-stimulatory and co-inhibitory factors, together making up the immune checkpoint (Table 2.1).[1,2] The activated T cell, via the T cell receptor (TCR), is an effector of the adaptive immune response, leading to B cell responses, macrophage activation and cytotoxic cell killing.[2]

It might be expected that tumour cells, with their diverse set of tumour-associated antigens acquired through genetic instability and epigenetic modification, would be easily recognized by the host immune system. Immune resistance through dysregulation of immune checkpoints is, however, commonplace, and leads to T cell exhaustion (Table 2.2) and, ultimately, deletion of tumour-specific T cells.[2] Generally, the co-stimulatory pathways that regulate T cell activation are not implicated in tumour immune resistance. By contrast, the co-inhibitory pathways that negatively regulate T cell effector functions are often overexpressed in tumour cells.[2]

Unlike many of the other signalling pathways targeted by cancer therapeutics, those activated by immune checkpoint proteins appear non-redundant, and there is often synergy of effect when multiple immune checkpoints are targeted.[1,2] This makes them a tantalizing drug target. Both single and combination immunotherapies ultimately aim to rescue exhausted T cells, restoring their cytotoxic function.

Current and future therapeutic targets

Cytotoxic T lymphocyte-associated protein 4

Identified in 1987, cytotoxic T lymphocyte-associated protein 4 (CTLA-4) (cluster of differentiation [CD] 152) is constitutively expressed on regulatory T cells but is inducible in other T cells after activation.[3] It is produced in response to CD28 stimulatory signalling via the TCR and, as such, functions to regulate the early stages of T cell activation in lymphoid organs, attenuating the activation signal.[3] Its expression is regulated by nuclear factor of activated T cells (NFAT) and forkhead box P3 (FOXP3).[3,4] CTLA-4 and CD28 share the same ligands on antigen-presenting cells (APCs), CD80 (B7-1) and CD86 (B7-2), although CTLA-4 has a much higher binding affinity for both.[4,5] Mouse knockout models show that animals lacking CTLA-4 have lethal systemic immune hyperactivation.[5]

Table 2.1 Checkpoints, ligands and therapeutic compounds (commercial and experimental) (adapted from Dempke et al.[1] and Pardoll[2]).

Checkpoint	Ligand	Role	Examples of therapeutic compounds
CTLA-4	CD80/CD86	Co-inhibitory	Ipilimumab, tremelimumab
PD-1	PD-L1/PD-L2	Co-inhibitory	Pembrolizumab, nivolumab, atezolizumab, avelumab, durvalumab
TIM-3	Galectin-9/HMGB1	Co-inhibitory	MGB453, TSR-022
LAG-3	MHC class II	Co-inhibitory	BMS-986016
TIGIT	CD155	Co-inhibitory	BMS-986207, MTIG7192A, OMP-313M32
VISTA	VISTAL (VSIG3)	Co-inhibitory	JNJ-61610588, CA-170
BTLA	HVEM	Co-inhibitory	NA
KIR	MHC class I	Co-inhibitory	Lirilumab
A2AR	Adenosine	Co-inhibitory	PBF-509, tozadenant, ST1535, ST4206, V81444
CD28	CD80/CD86	Co-stimulatory	TGN1412
ICOS	ICOSL/B7RP1	Co-stimulatory	JTX-2011
CD137	CD137L	Co-stimulatory	Utomilumab
GITR	GITRL	Co-stimulatory	TRX518-001
CD27	CD70	Co-stimulatory	Varlilumab
OX40	OX40L	Co-stimulatory	MOXR0916
CD40	CD40L	Co-stimulatory	CP-870,893
CD122	Not known	Co-stimulatory	NKTR-214
CD137	CD137L	Co-stimulatory	Lipocalin (bi-specific for HER2)

A2AR, adenosine A_{2A} receptor; BTLA, B and T lymphocyte attenuator; GITR, glucocorticoid-induced tumour necrosis factor receptor-related protein; HER2, human epidermal growth factor receptor 2; HVEM, herpes virus entry mediator; ICOS, inducible co-stimulatory molecule; KIR, killer-cell immunoglobulin-like receptor; OX40, tumour necrosis factor receptor superfamily, member 4; VISTA, V-domain immunoglobulin-containing suppressor of T cell activation.

CTLA-4 competes with CD28 for CD80 and CD86 binding, and also inhibits interleukin (IL)-2 secretion by T cells. CTLA-4 is thought to attenuate T cell activation by recruitment of a key phosphatase, Src homology region 2-containing protein tyrosine phosphatase (SHP)-2, ultimately leading to TCR dephosphorylation in a phosphoinositide 3-kinase (PI3K)-dependent mechanism (Figure 2.1).[1,2] CTLA-4 may also function by 'capturing' CD80 and CD86 from cell membranes, making them unavailable for CD28-dependent stimulation. Supporting this, CD28 had been shown to localize only to the T cell plasma membrane, whereas CTLA-4 may also be found in the endosomal compartment.[3]

Table 2.2 Role of co-inhibitory signals and cytokine production in T cell exhaustion. Upregulation of co-inhibitory pathways, with correlating patterns of cytokine production, leads to a stepwise loss of cytotoxic function and progression of the 'exhausted' phenotype. Severely exhausted T cells are eventually targeted for apoptosis and are therefore deleted from the host immune repertoire.[1–3,7]

Factor	Progressive T cell exhaustion				
IL-2	++	+	–	–	–
TNF-α	+++	+	–	–	–
IFN-γ	+++	++	+	–	–
PD-1	–	++	+++	+++	+++
TIM-3	–	++	+++	+++	+++
LAG-3	–	++	+++	++	++
Cytotoxicity	+++	++	+/–	–	–
Proliferation	+++	++	+	–	–
Apoptosis	–	–	+/–	++	+++

IFN-γ, interferon-γ; TNF-α, tumour necrosis factor-α.

The anti-CTLA-4 monoclonal antibody ipilimumab is approved for the treatment of locally advanced and metastatic melanoma. An immunoglobulin G1 monoclonal antibody, it binds CTLA-4 via a VH and VL segment-specific mechanism and also mediates antibody-dependent cellular cytotoxicity and complement-dependent cytotoxicity via its Fc portion.[6]

Programmed cell death protein 1

Programmed cell death protein 1 (PD-1) (CD279), first cloned in 1992, acts at a later stage than CTLA-4 in the immune response, limiting the activity of mature T cells in peripheral tissues to prevent an exaggerated immune response. It is also expressed on B cells, activated APCs and natural killer (NK) tumour-infiltrating lymphocytes (TILs).[2]

Pdcd1 knockout mice do not display embryonic lethality but do develop indolent autoimmune diseases, which supports this later stage role.[2] It also mirrors the clinical picture, where immune-related adverse events are more common and often higher grade with anti-CTLA-4 antibodies than with anti-PD-1 therapies.[1,2]

When engaged with its ligand, PD-1 is thought to act in an SHP-2-dependent manner, inhibiting PI3K signalling and downregulating T cell activation (Figure 2.1).[1,2] Recently, however, it has been postulated that the true target of the PD-1–SHP-2 complex may be CD28.[7] PD-1 ligands include programmed death-ligand 1 (PD-L1) (expressed on tumour cells and immune cells) and programmed death-ligand 2 (PD-L2) (expressed on dendritic cells of normal tissue, especially lung). PD-L1 has been shown to interact with CD80, making it unavailable for CD28 co-stimulation, while PD-L2 interacts with repulsive guidance molecule B (RGMb), with a function in respiratory tolerance.[1,2,7]

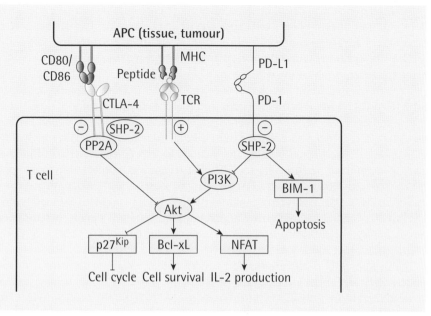

Figure 2.1 T cell activation and co-inhibition. T cell activation is initiated by recognition of peptide antigens presented by APCs to the TCR. Co-stimulation is provided by CD28 (not shown). Once activated, co-inhibitory pathways are upregulated to attenuate activation. CTLA-4 and PD-1 both function to inhibit protein kinase B (Akt) activation, by independent mechanisms but both employing SHP-2. CTLA-4 functions through the Ser/Thr protein phosphatase 2 (PP2A). PD-1 functions through the PI3K pathway. In addition, PD-1 ligation also signals through the Ras/Raf/mitogen-activated protein kinase kinase (MEK)/ERK/MAPK pathway to upregulate the proapoptotic molecule bisindolylmaleimide 1 (BIM-1). Bcl-xL, B cell lymphoma–extra large; p27[Kip], cyclin-dependent kinase inhibitor.[1,2]

There are several anti-PD-1 and anti-PD-L1 monoclonal antibodies currently available commercially, with an array of indications. The mechanisms of drug–receptor binding remain poorly elucidated. Crystallographic studies suggest that pembrolizumab and nivolumab, both V segment-dependent immunoglobulin G4 antibodies, bind to independent sites on PD-1, with no overlap.[8] Unsurprisingly, there is also a degree of structural homology between these two PD-1 drug-binding epitopes and PD-L1. Unlike CTLA-4, there is no evidence of Fc-mediated antibody-dependent cellular cytotoxicity activity.[8]

Emerging therapeutic checkpoint targets

A second wave of immune checkpoints are gaining clinical momentum. Lymphocyte-activation gene (LAG)-3 protein (CD223), first characterized in 1990, has high structural homology to CD4. Expressed on activated T cells and NK cells, it is thought to have a role in regulatory T cell-suppressive function and is often found co-expressed with PD-1 on TILs.[9] Its major ligand is major histocompatibility complex (MHC) class II, to which it binds with a much higher affinity compared with CD4.[9] By competitive inhibition of CD4/TCR interactions, LAG-3 limits overactivation and prevents the onset of autoimmunity. Persistent antigen exposure in the tumour microenvironment results, however, in sustained LAG-3 expression and T cell exhaustion (Figure 2.1).[1,2]

In keeping with this, *Lag3* knockout mice are phenotypically normal under unstressed conditions but show uncontrolled T cell expansion when challenged.[9] Two further LAG-3 ligands have been described: LSECtin and galectin-3 both inhibit the anti-tumour T cell response.[9] Several LAG-3 antibodies are currently in early phase clinical studies, including BMS-986016, which is being trialled in combination with the anti-PD-1 antibody nivolumab in melanoma.

T cell immunoglobulin and mucin domain (TIM)-3 (CD366; hepatitis A virus cellular receptor 2 [HAVCR2]) was described in 2002 and is a negative modulator of type 1 autoimmunity.[9,10] It is found on CD4+ cells and tumour antigen-specific CD8+ T cells, and is also expressed on regulatory T cells, NK and dendritic cells. Like all members of the TIM family, TIM-3 has a role in apoptosis.[10] Four ligand-binding interactions have been characterized. Binding to galectin-9 leads to an influx of calcium ions into Th1 cells, triggering apoptosis. Binding to phosphatidylserine leads to cells being marked for scavenging by phagocytes.[10] Where there is an abundance of nucleic acids (e.g. from apoptosing tumour cells), TIM-3 competes for high mobility group box 1 (HMGB1) binding to inhibit the innate immune system.[10] Finally, heterodimeric binding to carcinoembryonic antigen-related cell adhesion molecule 1 (CEACAM1) has been shown to act as a negative regulator of T cell responses.[10]

The degree of TIM-3 expression on cancer cells correlates with a rapid disease course and shorter survival. There are currently at least two anti-TIM-3 monoclonal antibodies in early phase clinical trials: MBG453 (ClinicalTrials.gov NCT02608268) and TSR-022 (ClinicalTrials.gov NCT02817633) are being trialled as monotherapy and alongside anti-PD-1 monoclonal antibodies in advanced malignancies.

T cell immunoreceptor with immunoglobulin and ITIM domains (TIGIT) was identified in 2009 by genome-wide screening for novel members of the CD28 superfamily.[9,11] Reminiscent of the CD28/CTLA-4 co-stimulant/co-inhibitory relationship, TIGIT shares a ligand (CD155) with the co-stimulatory receptor CD226, TIGIT having the higher binding affinity. TIGIT has also been shown to be able to directly bind to CD226 in mouse models, and as such also has a potential co-stimulatory mechanism of action.[11]

Dendritic cell CD155 binding by TIGIT influences the balance of cytokine production and leads to tolerance. Upon binding, TIGIT becomes phosphorylated, recruiting SHP-1, which leads to signal transduction blockade of both PI3K and mitogen-activated protein kinase (MAPK) (extracellular signal-regulated kinase [ERK] and p38) pathways, limiting nuclear factor κB (NFκB) signalling and leading to NK cell inhibition.[11] TIGIT has also been shown to directly induce T cell inhibition by targeting the TCR-signalling pathway, downregulating constituents of the TCR complex.

There are at least three anti-TIGIT monoclonal antibodies in early phase trials for advanced solid malignancies: BMS-986207 (ClinicalTrials.gov NCT02913313), MTIG7192A (ClinicalTrials.gov NCT02794571 and NCT03563716) and OMP-313M32 (ClinicalTrials.gov NCT03119428) are being investigated as monotherapies and in combination with anti-PD-1/anti-PD-L1/anti-PD-L2 agents.

Combination checkpoint therapy

Preclinical data strongly support the concept of synergistic interaction when independent immune checkpoints are inhibited, usually via enhanced immune function. At present only one combination has been approved by the US Food and Drug Administration (FDA): the PD-1 inhibitor nivolumab with the anti-CTLA-4 molecule ipilimumab. Based on the results of the phase II trial CheckMate 069, which saw a response rate of 60% for the combination, with 17% achieving a complete radiological response, vs an 11% response rate for ipilimumab alone (and no complete responses), the combination received FDA accelerated approved for the treatment of *BRAF* wild-type metastatic melanoma. As might have been predicted, however, there were far more grades 3–4 adverse events in patients in the combination arm (54% vs 20%, leading to 30% in combination arm patients who discontinued treatment) than in patients in the single-agent ipilimumab arm (9%).[12]

Conclusion

 Our understanding of cancer immunotherapy is in its infancy, and much is based on the better characterized pathways, CTLA-4 and PD-1. Existing biomarkers for patient selection, for example tumour PD-L1 expression, are suboptimal, reflecting the limitations of our knowledge.

Even in the biomarker unselected population, immune checkpoint blockade has a durable clinical benefit in a proportion of patients, reflecting that PD-1/PD-L1 pathway inhibition results in functional restoration of exhausted cytotoxic T cells. Combination immunotherapy may result in synergistic effects, further enhancing this effect; the addition of anti-CTLA-4 agents is already standard of care in metastatic melanoma. The effects of targeting novel targets such as TIM-3, LAG-3 and TIGIT are being explored both as mono- and combination therapy.

Elucidating the mechanism of action of ICPIs and their effects on the tumour immune environment will result in treatments tailored to an individual's specific cancer immunosignature, creating personalized regimens that maximize the chances of a durable clinical benefit.

References

1   Dempke WCM, Fenchel K, Uciechowski P, Dale SP. Second- and third-generation drugs for immune-oncology treatment. The more the better? *Eur J Cancer* 2017; 74: 55–72.

2   Pardoll DM. The blockade of immune checkpoints in cancer immunotherapy. *Nat Rev Cancer* 2012; 12: 252–64.

3   Wolchok JD, Saenger Y. The mechanism of anti-CTLA-4 activity and the negative regulation of T-cell activation. *Oncologist* 2008; 13 (suppl 4): 2–9.

4   Lee KM, Chuang E, Griffin M, *et al*. Molecular basis of T cell inactivation by CTLA-4. *Science* 1998; 282: 2263–6.

5   Schildberg FA, Klein SR, Freeman GJ, Sharpe AH. Coinhibitory pathways in the B7-CD28 ligand-receptor family. *Immunity* 2016; 44: 955–72.

6   He M, Chai Y, Qi J, *et al*. Remarkably similar CTLA-4 binding properties of therapeutic ipilimumab and tremelimumab antibodies. *Oncotarget* 2017; 8: 67129–39.

7   Hui E, Cheung J, Zhu J, *et al*. T cell costimulatory receptor CD28 is a primary target for PD-1 mediated inhibition. *Science* 2017; 355: 1428–33.

8   Fessas P, Lee H, Ikemizu S, Janowitz T. A molecular and preclinical comparison of the PD-1 targeted T-cell checkpoint inhibitors nivolumab and pembrolizumab. *Semin Oncol* 2017; 44: 136–40.

9   Anderson AC, Joller N, Kuchroo VK. Lag-3, Tim-3, and TIGIT: co-inhibitory receptors with specialized functions in immune regulation. *Immunity* 2016; 44: 989–1004.

10 Du W, Yang M, Turner A, *et al*. Tim-3 as a target for cancer immunotherapy and mechanisms of action. *Int J Mol Sci* 2017; 18: 645–57.

11 Manieri NA, Chiang EY, Grogan JL. TIGIT: a key inhibitor of the cancer immunity cycle. *Trends Immunol* 2017; 38: 20–8.

12 Hodi FS, Chesney J, Pavlick AC, *et al*. Combined nivolumab and ipilimumab versus ipilimumab alone in patients with advanced melanoma: 2-year overall survival outcomes in a multicentre, randomised, controlled, phase 2 trial. *Lancet Oncol* 2016; 17: 1558–68.

03 Immune Checkpoint Inhibitors: Successes and Challenges

Elizabeth Appleton, Christy Ralph

Introduction

The last 20 years have signalled a dramatic change in the clinical landscape of cancer therapeutics. Since the early 1990s, when interleukin (IL)-2, a T cell growth factor, first gained US Food and Drug Administration approval for the treatment of kidney cancer and melanoma, there has been a rising tide of immunotherapy. The field continues to attract vast scientific, clinical, patient and public attention; a Google search of 'cancer immunotherapy' yields over 2 million results, and there are thousands of ongoing clinical trials worldwide.

Undoubtedly the biggest change in this field in recent years has been the advent of immune checkpoint inhibitors (ICPIs). The immune checkpoints are a network of stimulatory and inhibitory receptors and ligands that are attractive as therapeutic targets because of their role in the regulation of the immune response. The upregulation of immune checkpoints such as cytotoxic T lymphocyte-associated protein 4 (CTLA-4), programmed cell death protein 1 (PD-1) and programmed death-ligand 1 (PD-L1) normally act to downregulate the immune response to chronic antigenic exposure.[1] These pathways may be exploited by cancer cells as they develop mechanisms to evade host immunity and thrive. The theory that blocking elements of these pathways has the potential to reverse tumour-induced immunosuppression and stimulate the immune system to eliminate cancer cells has led to a flood of scientific and clinical research.

Successes

In 2010, Hodi *et al.*[2] published a pivotal phase III trial demonstrating efficacy of the first ICPI in advanced melanoma. The agent was ipilimumab, an immunoglobulin G1 monoclonal antibody targeting CTLA-4. Ipilimumab was shown to prolong overall survival (OS) (10.1 vs 6.4 months, HR 0.68, $p<0.001$) in patients with pretreated advanced melanoma, achieving an overall response rate of 10.9%. Response was seen to be independent of common predictors of outcome (age, sex, stage, lactate dehydrogenase [LDH] level, prior high-dose IL-2).[2]

Despite the low and unpredictable response rate and significant toxicity (grades 3–4 in 10–15% of patients), the demonstration of a survival advantage signalled a revolution in the treatment of advanced melanoma.[2] A pooled analysis of long-term survival data showed a proportion of durable responses to treatment, with around 20% of patients surviving 3 years:[3] a striking contrast to the historically poor prognosis of these patients.

Since this seminal study, research into checkpoint-targeted immunotherapeutic agents has grown exponentially in a variety of cancer types. In what is often termed a 'gold rush' approach to clinical research, the efficacy of these targeted agents has been assessed across a broad range of solid and haematological malignancies in recent years. The rate of change and volume of research in this field are astounding, and any attempt to comprehensively summarize them would risk becoming rapidly obsolete. This chapter reviews recent research and highlights some key developments and emerging patterns of response.

Many indications and agents have shown significant promise. In 2015, the KEYNOTE-006 study in patients with advanced melanoma achieved better results on all counts with the anti-PD-1 receptor agent pembrolizumab compared with single-agent ipilimumab: response rates were higher (34% vs 11.9%), 12 month survival was better (68–74% vs 58%), and there were fewer serious toxic adverse events (10.9–13.1% vs 19.9%).[4] Ongoing evaluation of survival data from this study continues to provide evidence of superiority. When the final OS data from the KEYNOTE-006 study were published in 2017, median survival in the ipilimumab group was 16.0 months but it had not yet been reached in the pembrolizumab treatment groups.[5] Pembrolizumab has also shown benefit in non-small-cell lung carcinoma (NSCLC) when compared with standard chemotherapy. KEYNOTE-024 found improvements in progression-free survival (PFS) (10.3 vs 6.7 months) and response rate (44.8% vs 27.8%) in patients with high PD-L1 expression (>50%).[6]

Nivolumab, another anti-PD-1 monoclonal antibody, has shown improved survival benefit in both metastatic renal clear cell cancer[7] and recurrent head and neck cancer, with a modest median improvement in OS of 2.4 months.[8]

These positive results heralded the new class of therapeutic agents as 'wonder drugs' in an era of change, with growing indications, both as single agents and in combination therapy, in lung, melanoma, head and neck cancer, lymphoma, renal cancer and more. Importantly, single-agent anti-PD-1 drugs have not only been shown to have superior efficacy compared with traditional cytotoxic chemotherapy, but significantly fewer toxicities are experienced. For example, in the CheckMate 024 study of pembrolizumab in NSCLC, treatment-related adverse events occurred in 73.4% of patients in the pembrolizumab group and in 90.0% of patients in the chemotherapy group. Grades 3–5 treatment-related adverse events occurred in twice as many patients in the chemotherapy group as in the pembrolizumab group (53.3% vs 26.6%).[6]

More recently, combination treatment of ipilimumab and nivolumab has built on the success of single-agent immunotherapy, most notably again in the treatment of metastatic melanoma. The CheckMate 067 study of combination ipilimumab plus nivolumab vs either drug as a single agent demonstrated that, at a minimum follow-up of 36 months, the median OS had not been reached in the nivolumab plus ipilimumab group, compared with 37.6 months in the nivolumab group and 19.9 months in the ipilimumab group (HR for death with nivolumab plus ipilimumab vs ipilimumab, 0.55 [$p<0.001$]; HR for death with nivolumab vs ipilimumab, 0.65 [$p<0.001$]). Three year OS rates were 58% in the combination group compared with 52% and 34% in the nivolumab and ipilimumab groups, respectively. Despite the increased toxicities experienced with combination ICPI therapy, long-term outcome data are awaited with anticipation.

There have, however, been disappointing results with ICPI studies in some other common cancers. Kwon et al.[9] demonstrated negative results when ipilimumab was compared with placebo in advanced prostate cancer, as has been the case with pancreatic and most colorectal cancers – sites often deemed to be less 'immunogenic'. It is notable that some of these studies reveal complex survival curves: the first few months see an increased HR for death with ICPIs compared with other approaches, a finding that does not seem to be fully explained by drug toxicity. There has been recent recognition that some patients may experience a 'hyper-progressive' phenomenon in response to ICPI treatment, but the frequency and predictive features are yet to be well characterized.[10]

Despite this, signals of response are sometimes apparent even in negative studies where some subgroups of patients do well. For example, exploratory analyses in a second negative phase III trial of ipilimumab in prostate cancer showed an improvement in PFS and prostate-specific antigen response.[11] A negative phase III trial evaluating the CTLA-4 targeted monoclonal antibody tremelimumab in melanoma showed some evidence of a durable response (35.8 months vs 13.7 for standard chemotherapy),[12] although it is unclear how many of these patients might have later been treated with other agents. A recent phase III trial of the PD-L1 inhibitor atezolizumab in bladder cancer did not meet its primary endpoint of improving OS despite promising results in phase II. The median duration of response has not yet been reached, however, in patients with high PD-L1 expression, suggesting there may be evidence of durability for some patients.[13] This highlights the complex and still poorly understood dynamic interaction between cancer and the immune system, along with some of the potential difficulties faced when designing clinical trials to identify signals of response to these novel agents rather than to standard cytotoxic chemotherapies.

Challenges

For those who benefit, ICPIs have a significant impact on survival in comparison with standard therapy. For clinicians and patients, these results are changing cancer treatment in poor prognosis disease with the small but real hope of durable benefit that may be measured in years rather than short months. Despite growing research, however, the identification of potential long-term responders and those at risk of novel and life-threatening toxicities remains a challenge. Also, clinicians have a responsibility to manage patients' and public expectations. The resulting media coverage broadly publicized the availability of these agents and has led to a degree of mismatch between the narrative in the public domain and the reality of treatment for many patients. Fewer than half of patients respond to single-agent immunotherapy, with modest survival benefits for the majority. For example, while a remarkable 22% of patients survive 3 years after ipilimumab treatment for advanced melanoma, median survival remains only 11.4 months, and 50% of patients die within the first year.[3] It is also often perceived that these new, targeted agents are more tolerable than traditional treatments. While this is true for many of these therapies, the potential toxicities from these agents are novel and may be wide ranging and potentially long lasting – a factor that becomes even more relevant when considering the proportion of 'non-responders'. It is not always clear that these drugs are of such benefit in the less fit, the elderly and those with other complex medical problems who tend to be excluded from registration studies but fill oncology clinics.

Reliable and practical predictive markers of response and toxicity would therefore be of great benefit to clinicians and patients. A rapid increase in pharmaceutical company interest fuelled by a huge financial market share (now nearly USD 9 billion) has increased capacity for large-scale clinical trials. As a result, clinical data and drug development have in many cases overtaken scientific research into markers of response and vulnerability. Some potential candidates to predict response include LDH level, which has been shown to correlate with treatment resistance to ipilimumab therapy; an increase in lymphocyte count during treatment has also been associated with better clinical efficacy.[14] Patients with a high mutational load (the number of somatic mutations in tumour cells) gained greater clinical benefit from ipilimumab and pembrolizumab treatment.[15] With the exception, however, of PD-L1 status in NSCLC, no marker has yet been developed and validated for widespread use.

These new drugs are expensive; in the UK, NICE undertakes a programme of formal technology appraisals balancing clinical and financial evidence before issuing guidance and recommendations about new medicines (Table 3.1). Safe delivery of ICPIs requires education of staff and changes to delivery and toxicity management services for patients. Cost and capacity will affect

Table 3.1 NICE-approved indications for use of ICPIs in non-haematological malignancies (July 2018).

Drug	Target	Indication	Dose and frequency	Phase III data	Toxicities	Cost per QALY gained
Ipilimumab	CTLA-4	Advanced melanoma, previously treated and untreated	3 mg/kg every 3 weeks	Median OS 10.1 months (HR 0.68, RR 10.9%)[2]	10–15% grades 3–4	£28,600–£47,900[16]
Pembrolizumab	PD-1	Advanced melanoma	2 mg/kg every 3 weeks	Results for 3 weekly regimen: estimated 12 month OS 68.4% (HR 0.69, RR 32.9%)[4]	10.1–13.1% grades 3–5	Confidential; ICER <£50,000[17]
Pembrolizumab	PD-1	Untreated PD-L1-positive metastatic NSCLC with no EGFR- or ALK-positive mutations	200 mg every 3 weeks	Median PFS 10.3 months (HR 0.50, RR 44.8%) Stopped at second interim analysis to allow crossover[6]	26.6% grades 3–5	£30,000–£50,000[18]
Pembrolizumab	PD-1	Previously treated metastatic PD-L1-positive NSCLC	2 mg/kg every 3 weeks	Median OS 10.4 months (HR 0.71)[19]	13% grades 3–5	£44,490–£61,954[20]
Pembrolizumab	PD-1	Advanced urothelial cancer; cisplatin unsuitable (in CDF)	200 mg every 3 weeks	Phase II: median OS 11.0 months[21]	16% grades 3–5	£43,702–£65,642[22]
Pembrolizumab	PD-1	Advanced urothelial cancer after platinum-based chemotherapy	200 mg every 3 weeks	Median OS 10.3 months vs 7.4 chemotherapy (HR 0.73, RR 21%) No change in PFS[23]	15% grades 3–5 vs 49.4%	£44,504–£46,447[24]
Nivolumab	PD-1	Advanced melanoma	3 mg/kg every 2 weeks	Median PFS 5.1 months (HR 0.43, RR 40%)[25]	11.7% grades 3–4	Confidential; ICER <£30,000[26]

Drug	Target	Indication	Dosing	Efficacy	Toxicity	Cost
Nivolumab	PD-1	Previously treated NSCLC (in CDF)	3 mg/kg every 2 weeks	Median OS 12.2 months (HR 0.71, RR 19%)[27]	10% grades 3–4	£50,014[28]
Nivolumab + ipilimumab	PD-1/CTLA-4	Advanced melanoma	Nivolumab 1 mg/kg + ipilimumab 3 mg/kg every 3 weeks for four doses, then nivolumab 3 mg/kg every 2 weeks	Median PFS 11.5 months (HR 0.42, RR 57.6%)[29]	55% grades 3–4	£29,900 (compared with pembrolizumab)[30]
Nivolumab	PD-1	Previously treated metastatic renal cell carcinoma	3 mg/kg every 2 weeks	Median OS 25 months (HR 0.73, RR 25%)[7]	19% grades 3–4	Confidential; ICER <£50,000[31]
Nivolumab	PD-1	Squamous cell head and neck cancer after platinum-based chemotherapy (in CDF)	3 mg/kg every 2 weeks	Median OS 7.5 months (HR 0.70, RR 13.3%)[8]	13.1% grades 3–4	£45,000–£58,500[32]
Atezolizumab	PD-L1	Advanced urothelial cancer after platinum-based chemotherapy (in CDF)	1200 mg every 3 weeks	Phase II: RR 15.8% Median OS 7.9 months[33]	20% grades 3–4	£100,844–£154,282; confidential arrangement led to CDF approval[34]
Atezolizumab	PD-L1	NSCLC after chemotherapy	1200 mg every 3 weeks	Median OS 13.8 months vs 9.6 HR 0.73[35]	15% grades 3–4	Confidential; no ICER released[36]

CDF, Cancer Drugs Fund; ICER, incremental cost-effectiveness ratio; QALY, quality-adjusted life year.

roll out of new treatments even when they are of proven clinical benefit. As a result, without international support and collaboration, safe and financially viable use of these drugs for the time being is only likely to be an option for patients in wealthier parts of the world. In addition, the increased duration and frequency of treatment, along with the wide range of short- and long-term toxicities, leads to increased patient contact time, hospital visits and admissions.

Conclusion

The advent of ICPI therapy represents an exciting era in cancer immunotherapy, with the potential for durable responses in those who would previously have had limited effective treatment options. The complex interplay between cancer and the immune system, however, means that predicting individual response and toxicity remains a challenge. More research is needed to manage the balance between growing demand and practical, effective service delivery.

References

1 Peggs KS, Quezada SA, Allison JP. Cancer immunotherapy: co-stimulatory agonists and co-inhibitory antagonists. *Clin Exp Immunol* 2009; 157: 9–19.

2 Hodi FS, O'Day SJ, McDermott DF, *et al*. Improved survival with ipilimumab in patients with metastatic melanoma. *N Engl J Med* 2010; 363: 711–23.

3 Schadendorf D, Hodi FS, Robert C, *et al*. Pooled analysis of long-term survival data from phase II and phase III trials of ipilimumab in unresectable or metastatic melanoma. *J Clin Oncol* 2015; 33: 1889–94.

4 Robert C, Schachter J, Long GV, *et al*. Pembrolizumab versus ipilimumab in advanced melanoma. *N Engl J Med* 2015; 372: 2521–32.

5 Schachter J, Ribas A, Long GV, *et al*. Pembrolizumab versus ipilimumab for advanced melanoma: final overall survival results of a multicentre, randomised, open-label phase 3 study (KEYNOTE-006). *Lancet* 2017; 390: 1853–62.

6 Reck M, Rodríguez-Abreu D, Robinson AG, *et al*. Pembrolizumab versus chemotherapy for PD-L1-positive non-small-cell lung cancer. *N Engl J Med* 2016; 375: 1823–33.

7 Motzer RJ, Escudier B, McDermott DF, *et al*. Nivolumab versus everolimus in advanced renal-cell carcinoma. *N Engl J Med* 2015; 373: 1803–13.

8 Ferris RL, Blumenschein G Jr, Fayette J, *et al*. Nivolumab for recurrent squamous-cell carcinoma of the head and neck. *N Engl J Med* 2016; 375: 1856–67.

9 Kwon ED, Drake CG, Scher HI, *et al*. Ipilimumab versus placebo after radiotherapy in patients with metastatic castration-resistant prostate cancer that had progressed after docetaxel chemotherapy (CA184–043): a multicentre, randomised, double-blind, phase 3 trial. *Lancet Oncol* 2014; 15: 700–12.

10 Champiat S, Dercle L, Ammari S, *et al*. Hyperprogressive disease is a new pattern of progression in cancer patients treated by anti-PD-1/PD-L1. *Clin Cancer Res* 2017; 23: 1920–8.

11 Beer TM, Kwon ED, Drake CG, *et al*. Randomized, double-blind, phase III trial of ipilimumab versus placebo in asymptomatic or minimally symptomatic patients with metastatic chemotherapy-naive castration-resistant prostate cancer. *J Clin Oncol* 2017; 35: 40–7.

12 Ribas A, Kefford R, Marshall MA, *et al.* Phase III randomized clinical trial comparing tremelimumab with standard-of-care chemotherapy in patients with advanced melanoma. *J Clin Oncol* 2013; 31: 616–22.

13 Cattrini C, Boccardo F. Atezolizumab and bladder cancer: facing a complex disease. *Lancet* 2018; 391: 305–6.

14 Gibney GT, Weiner LM, Atkins MB. Predictive biomarkers for checkpoint inhibitor-based immunotherapy. *Lancet Oncol* 2016; 17: e542–51.

15 Manson G, Norwood J, Marabelle A, *et al.* Biomarkers associated with checkpoint inhibitors. *Ann Oncol* 2016; 27: 1199–206.

16 NICE (2014). *Ipilimumab for previously untreated advanced (unresectable or metastatic) melanoma. Technology appraisal guidance TA319.* Available from: www.nice.org.uk/guidance/ta319/chapter/4-Consideration-of-the-evidence (accessed 20 July 2018).

17 NICE (2015; updated 2017). *Pembrolizumab for treating advanced melanoma after disease progression with ipilimumab. Technology appraisal guidance TA357.* Available from: www.nice.org.uk/guidance/ta357/chapter/4-Consideration-of-the-evidence (accessed 20 July 2018).

18 NICE (2018). *Pembrolizumab for untreated PD-L1-positive metastatic non-small-cell lung cancer. Technology appraisal guidance TA531.* Available from: www.nice.org.uk/guidance/ta531/chapter/3-Committee-discussion#cost-effectiveness (accessed 20 July 2018).

19 Herbst RS, Baas P, Kim DW, *et al.* Pembrolizumab versus docetaxel for previously treated, PD-L1-positive, advanced non-small-cell lung cancer (KEYNOTE-010): a randomised controlled trial. *Lancet* 2016; 387: 1540–50.

20 NICE (2017). *Pembrolizumab for treating PD-L1-positive non-small-cell lung cancer after chemotherapy. Technology appraisal guidance TA428.* Available from: www.nice.org.uk/guidance/ta428/chapter/4-Committee-discussion (accessed 20 July 2018).

21 Balar AV, Castellano D, O'Donnell PH, *et al.* First-line pembrolizumab in cisplatin-ineligible patients with locally advanced and unresectable or metastatic urothelial cancer (Keynote-052): a multicentre, single-arm, phase 2 study. *Lancet Oncol* 2017; 18: 1483–92.

22 NICE (2018). *Pembrolizumab for untreated PD-L1-positive locally advanced or metastatic urothelial cancer when cisplatin is unsuitable. Technology appraisal guidance TA522.* Available from: www.nice.org.uk/guidance/ta522/chapter/3-Committee-discussion (accessed 20 July 2018).

23 Bellmunt J, de Wit R, Vaughn DJ, *et al.* Pembrolizumab as second-line therapy for advanced urothelial carcinoma. *N Engl J Med* 2017; 376: 1015–26.

24 NICE (2018). *Pembrolizumab for treating locally advanced or metastatic urothelial carcinoma after platinum-containing chemotherapy. Technology appraisal guidance TA519.* Available from: www.nice.org.uk/guidance/ta519/chapter/3-Committee-discussion (accessed 20 July 2018).

25 Weber JS, D'Angelo SP, Minor D, *et al.* Nivolumab versus chemotherapy in patients with advanced melanoma who progressed after anti-CTLA-4 treatment (CheckMate 037): a randomised, controlled, open-label, phase 3 trial. *Lancet Oncol* 2015; 16: 375–84.

26 NICE (2016). *Nivolumab for treating advanced (unresectable or metastatic) melanoma. Technology appraisal guidance TA384.* Available from: www.nice.org.uk/guidance/ta384/chapter/4-Committee-discussion (accessed 20 July 2018).

27   Horn L, Spigel DR, Vokes EE, *et al*. Nivolumab versus docetaxel in previously treated patients with advanced non-small-cell lung cancer: two-year outcomes from two randomized, open-label, phase III trials (CheckMate 017 and CheckMate 057). *J Clin Oncol* 2017; 35: 3924–33.

28   NICE (2017). *Nivolumab for previously treated squamous non-small-cell lung cancer. Technology appraisal guidance TA483*. Available from: www.nice.org.uk/guidance/ta483/chapter/4-Committee-discussion (accessed 20 July 2018).

29   Larkin J, Hodi FS, Wolchok JD. Combined nivolumab and ipilimumab or monotherapy in untreated melanoma. *N Engl J Med* 2015; 373: 1270–1.

30   NICE (2016). *Nivolumab in combination with ipilimumab for treating advanced melanoma. Technology appraisal guidance TA400*. Available from: www.nice.org.uk/guidance/ta400/chapter/4-Committee-discussion (accessed 20 July 2018).

31   NICE (2016; updated 2017). *Nivolumab for previously treated advanced renal cell carcinoma. Technology appraisal guidance TA417*. Available from: www.nice.org.uk/guidance/ta417/chapter/4-Committee-discussion (accessed 20 July 2018).

32   NICE (2017). *Nivolumab for treating squamous cell carcinoma of the head and neck after platinum-based chemotherapy. Technology appraisal guidance TA490*. Available from: www.nice.org.uk/guidance/ta490/chapter/3-Committee-discussion (accessed 20 July 2018).

33   Rosenberg JE, Hoffman-Censits J, Powles T, *et al*. Atezolizumab in patients with locally advanced and metastatic urothelial carcinoma who have progressed following treatment with platinum-based chemotherapy: a single-arm, multicentre, phase 2 trial. *Lancet* 2016; 387: 1909–20.

34   NICE (2018). *Atezolizumab for treating locally advanced or metastatic urothelial carcinoma after platinum-containing chemotherapy. Technology appraisal guidance TA525*. Available from: www.nice.org.uk/guidance/ta525/chapter/3-Committee-discussion (accessed 20 July 2018).

35   Rittmeyer A, Barlesi F, Waterkamp D, *et al*. Atezolizumab versus docetaxel in patients with previously treated non-small-cell lung cancer (OAK): a phase 3, open-label, multicentre randomised controlled trial. *Lancet* 2017; 389: 255–65.

36   NICE (2018). *Atezolizumab for treating locally advanced or metastatic non-small-cell lung cancer after chemotherapy. Technology appraisal guidance TA520*. Available from: www.nice.org.uk/guidance/ta520/chapter/3-Committee-discussion (accessed 20 July 2018).

04 Immune-Related Toxicity of Checkpoint Inhibitors

Lewis Au, James Clark, Jennifer Thomas, James Larkin

Introduction

Monoclonal antibodies targeting the immune checkpoint proteins cytotoxic T lymphocyte-associated protein 4 (CTLA-4), programmed cell death protein 1 (PD-1) and programmed death-ligand 1 (PD-L1) have shown significant efficacy in the treatment of multiple tumour types. Ipilimumab (anti-CTLA-4), pembrolizumab and nivolumab (anti-PD-1), as well as atezolizumab and durvalumab (anti-PD-L1), are lead examples of these agents. The trade-off for clinical activity of immune checkpoint inhibitors (ICPIs) is the potential for immune-related adverse events (irAEs). These are well-recognized complications of ICPIs and are also a significant cause of discontinuation of therapy and patient morbidity. The onset of irAEs is largely unpredictable in timing and may affect any organ in the body; there is currently a lack of clinical phenotype or biomarkers that reliably predict those who are destined to develop irAEs. Examples of irAEs range from mild reactions such as pruritus and skin rash, generally manageable on an outpatient basis, to more severe and clinically significant toxicities such as colitis, hepatitis and pneumonitis, which may lead to prolonged hospitalization. Furthermore, potentially fatal fulminant myocarditis and neurotoxicities may occur. All irAEs should be graded according to the Common Terminology Criteria for Adverse Events. Most toxicities are reversible with prompt institution of corticosteroids. Patients who develop immune-related endocrinopathies such as hypothyroidism, hypopituitarism and diabetes, however, are likely to require hormone replacement therapies indefinitely.

Rates of irAEs: agent, dosage, regimen and pre-existing autoimmunity

The expected rates of irAEs may be related to agent and dosage, and whether the ICPI is given as a combination regimen.

Ipilimumab was the first ICPI with proven efficacy for treatment of advanced cancer in the context of melanoma[1,2] and subsequently also in the adjuvant setting.[3] Ipilimumab dosed at 3 mg/kg for four doses every 3 weeks for the treatment of advanced melanoma has a drug-related toxicity rate of ~80%;[1] grades 3–4 irAEs were seen in ~30% of patients.[2] In the adjuvant setting, where ipilimumab was dosed at 10 mg/kg for four doses every 3 weeks, then every 3 months for up to 3 years, irAE rates of all grades were ~90%, and ~40% were grades 3–4.[3,4] A previous phase III study comparing ipilimumab dosed at 10 mg/kg vs 3 mg/kg for four doses every 3 weeks,[4] as well as a dose-ranging phase II study, supported the finding of increasing toxicities with escalating doses.[5] It is worthwhile noting that ipilimumab has been superseded both as standard initial therapy for advanced disease and in the adjuvant setting for the treatment of melanoma.

Treatment with single-agent anti-PD-1/anti-PD-L1 is generally well tolerated, and this is consistent across tumour types and approved treatment settings. Anti-PD-1 agents have been evaluated in phase III studies for advanced melanoma,[6] renal cell carcinoma,[7] non-small-cell lung carcinoma (NSCLC)[8] and recurrent squamous cell carcinoma of the head and neck[9] in the advanced setting. Rates of grades 3–4 irAEs of 11.7%, 19%, 10% and 13.1%, respectively, were recorded in these studies. Anti-PD-L1 agents have been used in NSCLC[10] and bladder cancer[11] in clinical trials. Rates of all grade irAEs were 24.2% and 12%, respectively, and rates of grades 3–4 irAEs were 8.1% and 7%, respectively, for durvalumab in NSCLC (phase III trial) and atezolizumab in bladder cancer (phase II trial).

In general, combination ICPI therapy is associated with higher rates of toxicity compared with monotherapy. Currently, combination ipilimumab (3 mg/kg every 3 weeks for four doses) plus nivolumab (1 mg/kg every 3 weeks for four doses, followed by 3 mg/kg every 2 weeks) is considered as a standard of care option for treatment of advanced melanoma, as evaluated in the Check-Mate 067 study.[12] In this phase III randomized trial of combination ipilimumab plus nivolumab vs each drug alone, the rate of grades 3–4 irAEs was reported to be 55%; 36% of patients treated in the combination arm discontinued therapy compared with 7.7% in the nivolumab arm and 14.8% in the ipilimumab arm. The renal phase III CheckMate 214 study evaluated a lower ipilimumab dosage regimen (1 mg/kg every 3 weeks for four doses) plus nivolumab (3 mg/kg every 3 weeks for four doses with ipilimumab, followed by nivolumab 3 mg/kg every 2 weeks) compared with sunitinib.[13] The authors reported a 17% rate of grades 3–4 irAEs in the ICPI arm. The outcome of the CheckMate 511 study (ClinicalTrials.gov NCT02714218) directly comparing ipilimumab (3 mg/kg) plus nivolumab (1 mg/kg) vs ipilimumab (1 mg/kg) plus nivolumab (3 mg/kg) in the advanced melanoma setting is awaited.

While there is a lack of reliable predictive biomarkers for development of irAEs, pre-existing autoimmune disorders may increase the risk of toxicities in ICPI therapies. The evidence for this comes mostly from retrospective studies. In a case series of 52 patients with pre-existing auto-immune diseases treated with anti-PD-1 monotherapy for advanced melanoma,[14] most patients (n=27) had rheumatological disorders and 20 patients (38%) experienced a flare of their autoimmune disease. This suggests a higher than expected irAE rate for single-agent PD-1. A smaller case series of 30 patients with autoimmune disease treated with ipilimumab has been published, in which 13 patients experienced significant exacerbation of their underlying autoimmunity.[15] There is limited published literature in this context for combination ICPI use.

Pattern and timing of irAEs

The profiles of irAEs are generally comparable across different ICPI agents: rash, diarrhoea/colitis, hepatitis and thyroid dysfunction are consistently dominant and clinically relevant features across ICPI studies. For advanced melanoma, where ICPIs have been most extensively studied, a pooled analysis of 576 patients who received single-agent nivolumab reported the following irAEs of any grade: skin (34%), gastrointestinal (13.4%), hypo/hyperthyroidism (6.3%), hepatic toxicity (4.2%).[16] In that study, 4% of patients experienced grades 3–4 irAEs. By comparison, another pooled analysis evaluated 448 patients who had received at least one dose of nivolumab 1 mg/kg plus ipilimumab 3 mg/kg every 3 weeks for four doses (induction phase) followed by nivolumab 3 mg/kg every 2 weeks (continuation phase) across phase I, II and III trials for melanoma.[17] The authors reported a rate of grades 3–4 irAEs of 55.4% for the study; all grade skin toxicity in 64.3% (grades 3–4 in 7.4%) was the most common irAE, followed by gastrointestinal (46%; grades 3–4, 16.3%), endocrine (29.7%; grades 3–4, 4.7%), hepatic (28.8%; grades 3–4, 17%) and pulmonary toxicity (7.6%; grades 3–4, 1.3%).

Regarding timing of presentation, irAEs may occur early (within 2 weeks of treatment)[17,18] or late (>12 months from start of therapy).[19] They may occur even after cessation of therapy. Median times to onset of toxicities were reported in pooled analyses by Weber *et al.*[16] and Sznol *et al.*[17] In these studies, median time to onset of any grade irAEs (for nivolumab) and grades 3–4 irAEs (for combination treatment) was within 12 weeks of starting therapy (Figures 4.1 and 4.2). This included skin, gastrointestinal, hepatic, endocrine and pulmonary toxicities. Most irAEs resolved within 6 weeks of therapy, with the exception of skin toxicities, which had a prolonged time to resolution (median 28.6 weeks for nivolumab). Endocrinopathies commonly required long-term hormone replacement therapy.

The rarer cardiac and neurological toxicities may present atypically and be fatal.[20,21] Rapidly progressive symptoms demand prompt action from the clinician. Clinicians should always maintain a high index of suspicion for irAEs in patients who have received ICPI treatment and present with variance from baseline symptoms.

General principles of irAE management

A high index of suspicion for immune-mediated pathology is required for any patient who develops new symptoms or laboratory abnormalities after ICPI treatment. Management is guided by both the organ system involved and its severity. At any grade, alternative aetiologies should be investigated and excluded through history, examination and appropriate investigations. Nevertheless, given the potential for irAEs to follow a fulminant course (particularly colitis, hepatitis, pneumonitis and myocarditis), immunosuppressive treatment should not be withheld for significant or worsening toxicities while awaiting further investigations. To date there are no

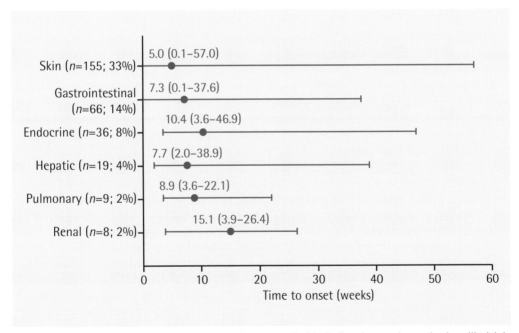

Figure 4.1 Time to onset of irAEs of any grade in patients treated with nivolumab monotherapy in phase III trials in melanoma (*n*=474). Shown are time to onset, number and incidence of irAEs. Circles represent median, bars denote range with values indicated above (adapted from Weber *et al.*[16]).

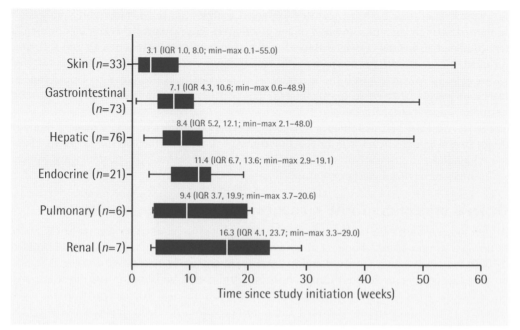

Figure 4.2 Time to onset of selected grades 3–4 irAEs with ipilimumab plus nivolumab in melanoma (*n*=448). Coloured boxes indicate interquartile range (IQR: Q1, Q3), central vertical line shows median, outer bars indicate range (values indicated above; minimum to maximum [min–max]) (adapted from Sznol *et al.*[17]).

randomized prospective studies to direct the management of irAEs. Guidelines such as those issued by the European Society for Medical Oncology[22] are based on multicentre experience and expert opinion consensus.

An example of organ system-specific management algorithms for common irAEs is described in Table 4.1. Broadly speaking, for gastrointestinal toxicity, ICPIs may be continued with supportive measures (such as mild topical steroids for skin rashes, or loperamide for diarrhoea) and vigilant surveillance. Patients should be counselled to report worsening symptoms and have a clear point of access to advice from experienced centres.

Treatment should usually be withheld during active grade 2 toxicity; the decision to initiate systemic steroids will depend on the organ system involved and on the duration and trajectory of symptoms. ICPI treatment may typically be restarted once toxicity has resolved and steroids have been weaned to a daily dose of no more than 10 mg prednisolone (or equivalent). For grade 3 or 4 toxicity affecting any organ, ICPIs should be withheld and high-dose systemic steroids initiated. If this does not lead to rapid improvement, early consideration should be given to the addition of further immunomodulatory agents such as tumour necrosis factor (TNF)-α antagonists, mycophenolate mofetil or tacrolimus. Patients should be managed in experienced centres with access to organ-specific multidisciplinary advice. On improvement, systemic steroids should be weaned gradually over weeks to months. Consideration of further ICPI treatment after resolution of toxicity requires careful analysis of risks and benefits and would rarely be considered after grade 4 events.

An important exception to this schema is immune-related endocrinopathy affecting the pituitary gland (hypophysitis), thyroid gland or endocrine pancreas. While systemic glucocorticoids

Table 4.1 Management of irAEs for selected grades 1–4 toxicities.

Organ system affected by irAE	Severity			
	Grade 1[a]	Grade 2[b]	Grade 3[c]	Grade 4[d]
Skin	Supportive management: topical emollients and oral antihistamines Continue ICPI	As per grade 1, plus moderate potency topical steroids Continue ICPI	Initiate systemic steroids: oral or intravenous (methyl)prednisolone 0.5–1 mg/kg per day Wean over 1–2 or 2–4 weeks according to severity Withhold ICPI until symptoms improve to grade 1 or mild grade 2	Initiate systemic steroids: intravenous methylprednisolone 1–2 mg/kg per day Permanently discontinue ICPI
Gastrointestinal	Symptomatic management: oral fluids, loperamide; avoid high-fibre/high-lactose diet If persists >14 days, treat as grade 2 Continue ICPI	As per grade 1, plus initiate steroids: oral prednisolone 0.5–1 mg/kg per day Withhold ICPI, but consider resuming treatment once symptoms have resolved; prednisolone ≤10 mg/kg per day	Initiate steroids: intravenous methylprednisolone 1–2 mg/kg per day If no improvement at 72 h or worsening, consider addition of infliximab 5 mg/kg Further immunosuppressive treatment options: mycophenolate mofetil 0.5–1 g twice daily, tacrolimus Permanently discontinue ICPI	
Hepatic	Continue ICPI	If ALT/AST rising when re-checked, consider oral prednisolone 1 mg/kg per day Withhold ICPI, but consider resuming once liver function tests normalize; prednisolone ≤10 mg/kg per day	Initiate steroids If ALT/AST ≤6.68 μkat/l and bilirubin/INR/albumin are normal: oral prednisolone 1 mg/kg per day If ALT/AST >6.68 μkat/l or bilirubin or INR is raised and albumin is low: intravenous methylprednisolone 2 mg/kg per day Withhold ICPI Re-challenge only at consultant's discretion	Initiate steroids: intravenous methylprednisolone 2 mg/kg per day Permanently discontinue ICPI
Pulmonary	Consider delaying ICPI	Initiate steroids: oral prednisolone 1 mg/kg per day Withhold ICPI	Initiate steroids: intravenous methylprednisolone 2–4 mg/kg per day If no improvement or worsening at 48 h, add infliximab 5 mg/kg Permanently discontinue ICPI	

[a]Grade 1, mild: asymptomatic or mild symptoms; clinical or diagnostic observations only; intervention not indicated.

[b]Grade 2, moderate: minimal, local or non-invasive intervention indicated; limiting instrumental activities of daily living.

[c]Grade 3, severe: hospitalization indicated; disabling; limiting self-care activities of daily living.

[d]Grade 4, life-threatening: urgent intervention indicated.

ALT, alanine aminotransferase; AST, aspartate aminotransferase; INR, international normalized ratio.

may be required to suppress inflammation in hypophysitis if there are features of mass effect such as headaches or neurological symptoms, timely immunosuppression does not appear to restore gland function. Management of endocrinopathy is generally through supportive measures and long-term hormone replacement. ICPI treatment should be withheld until recovery from symptoms, but may typically be restarted once patients are asymptomatic and stable on appropriate replacement.

Where patients require long courses of high-dose steroids for management of irAEs, care should be taken to minimize the risks of opportunistic infection with *Pneumocystis jirovecii* pneumonia. Gastro-protection with proton pump inhibition is recommended; consideration should be given to the impact on bone health, myopathy, mood and glycaemic control.

irAEs and treatment efficacy outcomes

Development and management of irAEs does not appear to compromise ICPI efficacy, although the evidence to date is limited to the setting of advanced melanoma. A pooled analysis of 409 patients treated with ipilimumab and nivolumab has shown similar progression-free and overall survival outcomes between patients who discontinued therapy because of adverse events compared with those who did not.[23] Similar results were reported in studies with ipilimumab-treated patients.[24] Other studies have suggested associations between the development of vitiligo and favourable clinical outcomes in the setting of advanced melanoma.[25,26]

Conclusion

While the use of ICPIs has revolutionized the treatment of an ever-expanding list of tumour types in various settings, better understanding and management of irAEs remains a critical area to address. The manifestations of irAEs may be diverse, and clinicians need to be vigilant when assessing patients who have received ICPIs. To date, there are no prospective studies evaluating the optimal strategy for management of organ-specific toxicities. Early recognition of irAEs and prompt administration of glucocorticoids for clinically significant irAEs remain the cornerstones of management. Treatment and development of irAEs do not appear to impact drug efficacy; however, more data are needed, particularly for various tumour types. Management of patients who develop irAEs in a multidisciplinary setting is critical in optimizing patient care.

References

1   Hodi FS, O'Day SJ, McDermott DF, *et al*. Improved survival with ipilimumab in patients with metastatic melanoma. *N Engl J Med* 2010; 363: 711–23.

2   Robert C, Thomas L, Bondarenko I, *et al*. Ipilimumab plus dacarbazine for previously untreated metastatic melanoma. *N Engl J Med* 2011; 364: 2517–26.

3   Eggermont AM, Chiarion-Sileni V, Grob JJ, *et al*. Adjuvant ipilimumab versus placebo after complete resection of high risk stage III melanoma (EORTC 18071): a randomised, double-blind, phase 3 trial. *Lancet Oncol* 2015; 16: 522–30.

4   Ascierto PA, Del Vecchio M, Robert C, *et al*. Ipilimumab 10 mg/kg versus ipilimumab 3 mg/kg in patients with unresectable or metastatic melanoma: a randomised, double-blind multicentre, phase 3 trial. *Lancet Oncol* 2017; 18: 611–22.

5   Weber J, Mandala M, Vechhio MD, *et al.* Adjuvant nivolumab versus ipilimumab in resected stage III or IV melanoma. *N Engl J Med* 2017; 377: 1824–35.

6   Robert C, Long GV, Dutriaux C, *et al.* Nivolumab in previously untreated melanoma without BRAF mutation. *N Engl J Med* 2015; 372: 320–30.

7   Motzer RJ, Escudier B, McDermott DF, *et al.* Nivolumab versus everolimus in advanced renal-cell carcinoma. *N Engl J Med* 2015; 373: 1803–13.

8   Borghaei H, Paz-Ares L, Horn L, *et al.* Nivolumab versus docetaxel in advanced non-squamous non-small-cell lung cancer. *N Engl J Med* 2015; 373: 1627–39.

9   Ferris RL, Blumenschein GJ, Fayette J, *et al.* Nivolumab for recurrent squamous-cell carcinoma of the head and neck. *N Engl J Med* 2016; 375: 1856–67.

10 Antonia SJ, Villegas A, Daniel D, *et al.* Furvalumab after chemoradiotherapy in stage III non-small-cell lung cancer. *N Engl J Med* 2017; 377: 1919–29.

11 Balar A, Galsky M, Rosenberg J, *et al.* Atezolizumab as first-line treatment in cisplatin-ineligible patients with locally advanced and metastatic urothelial carcinoma: a single-arm multicentre, phase 2 trial. *Lancet* 2016; 298: 67–76.

12 Larkin J, Chiarion-Sileni V, González R, *et al.* Combined nivolumab and ipilimumab or monotherapy in untreated melanoma. *N Engl J Med* 2015; 373: 23–34.

13 Motzer RJ, Tannir NM, McDermott DF, *et al.* Nivolumab plus ipilimumab versus sunitinib in advanced renal-cell carcinoma. *N Engl J Med* 2018; 378: 1277–90.

14 Menzies AM, Johnson DB, Ramanujam S, *et al.* Anti-PD-1 therapy in patients with advanced melanoma and preexisting autoimmune disorders or major toxicity with ipilimumab. *Ann Oncol* 2017; 28: 368–76.

15 Johnson DB, Sullivan RJ, Ott PA, *et al.* Ipilimumab therapy in patients with advanced melanoma and preexisting autoimmune disorders. *JAMA Oncol* 2016; 2: 234–40.

16 Weber JS, Hodi FS, Wolchok JD, *et al.* Safety profile of nivolumab monotherapy: a pooled analysis of patients with advanced melanoma. *J Clin Oncol* 2017; 35: 785–92.

17 Sznol M, Ferrucci PF, Hogg D, *et al.* Pooled analysis safety profile of nivolumab and ipilimumab combination therapy in patients with advanced melanoma. *J Clin Oncol* 2017; 35: 3815–22.

18 Weber JS, Kahler KC, Hauschild A. Management of immune-related adverse events and kinetics of response with ipilimumab. *J Clin Oncol* 2012; 30: 2691–7.

19 Naidoo J, Wang X, Woo KM, *et al.* Pneumonitis in patients treated with anti-programmed death-1/programmed death ligand 1 therapy. *J Clin Oncol* 2017; 35: 709–17.

20 Johnson DB, Balko JM, Compton ML, *et al.* Fulminant myocarditis with combination immune checkpoint blockade. *N Engl J Med* 2016; 375: 1749–55.

21 Eggermont AM, Chiarion-Sileni V, Grob JJ, *et al.* Adjuvant ipilimumab versus placebo after complete resection of high-risk stage III melanoma (EORTC 18071): a randomised, double-blind, phase 3 trial. *Lancet Oncol* 2015; 16: 522–30.

22 Haanen JBAG, Carbonnel F, Robert C, *et al.* Management of toxicities from immunotherapy: ESMO clinical practice guidelines for diagnosis, treatment and follow-up. *Ann Oncol* 2017; 28 (suppl 4): iv119–42.

23 Schadendorf D, Wolchok JD, Hodi FS, *et al.* Efficacy and safety outcomes in patients with advanced melanoma who discontinued treatment with nivolumab and ipilimumab because of adverse events: a pooled analysis of randomized phase II and III trials. *J Clin Oncol* 2017; 35: 3807–14.

24 Horvat TZ, Adel NG, Dang TO, *et al.* Immune-related adverse events, need for systemic immunosuppression, and effects on survival and time to treatment failure in patients with melanoma treated with ipilimumab at Memorial Sloan Kettering Cancer Center. *J Clin Oncol* 2015; 33: 3193–8.

25 Hua C, Boussemart L, Mateus C, *et al.* Association of vitiligo with tumor response in patients with metastatic melanoma treated with pembrolizumab. *JAMA Dermatol* 2016; 152: 45–51.

26 Teulings HE, Limpens J, Jansen SN, *et al.* Vitiligo-like depigmentation in patients with stage III–IV melanoma receiving immunotherapy and its association with survival: a systematic review and meta-analysis. *J Clin Oncol* 2015; 33: 773–81.

PERSPECTIVE

05 Predicting Response to Immunotherapy

Ioannis Karydis, Ruth E. Board

Introduction

The arrival of immunomodulatory agents has led to a paradigm shift in oncological practice. Immune checkpoint blockers such as nivolumab and ipilimumab have become standard of care in many malignancies, offering good chances of durable responses. The field of immuno-oncology is expanding rapidly and many dozens of immuno-oncological agents targeting distinct molecular pathways are currently in clinical trials.

Significant limitations remain, however: severe immune-related toxicity affects more than 50% of patients receiving combination ipilimumab/nivolumab regimens; a minority of patients may experience 'hyperprogression' in response to immunotherapy; the costs of these agents are not insignificant despite response rates in most tumour types being in the region of 15–30% for single agents.

Using combination regimens may improve efficacy, but in practical and financial terms it is not feasible to test each possible combination for every indication in unselected groups of patients. Preclinical studies to narrow down the field are challenging; the human immune system has marked differences even from that of closely related primate species, and animal models have repeatedly proven inadequate to predict clinical efficacy and toxicity.

Being able to predict which patients are more likely to respond to specific immunomodulatory approaches and how likely they are to experience specific side effects would alleviate these issues. This is the holy grail of current research in the field of immuno-oncology.

Challenges in developing biomarkers for tumour immunotherapy

Attempts at empirically discovering measurable indicators using peripheral blood have thus far failed to deliver usable biomarkers. One likely reason is that the crucial immune events take place in or adjacent to the cancer tissue. The picture derived from peripheral blood may bear very little resemblance to what is happening in the cancer tissue and may completely miss crucial cell populations such as tissue-resident memory T cells. Additionally, identifying peripheral blood-based proxy markers for events in the tumour microenvironment is extremely challenging without a good understanding of the underlying immune mechanisms.

To rectify this problem, access to suitable biopsy samples at critical time points is essential. This is not trivial to arrange and until recently was not routinely part of clinical trial design; moreover, in many tumour types access to tumour tissue is difficult at best and poses additional risks of biopsy-related discomfort and morbidity.

Recent developments in genomic, transcriptomic and proteomic techniques are rapidly expanding our knowledge of individual cell types, molecules and pathways involved in the human immune system. At the same time they expose critical gaps in our understanding of the complex networks involved. Despite advances in bioinformatics, building a complete model is beyond our current capabilities and limits our ability to rationally design predictive biomarkers for use of immuno-oncological agents.

Finally, enthusiasm among pharmaceutical companies has led to the parallel development of multiple immuno-oncological agents targeting the same pathways with matched diagnostic tests. Unfortunately, standardization is lacking in the techniques and methods used by different teams, making comparison or aggregation of results from multiple studies difficult if not impossible.

One way to address these issues is to fall back on basic principles. An effective anti-tumour immune response requires the following three elements:

- immune targets: tumour cells that either present peptides to which the host immune system has not been tolerized (i.e. neo- or cryptoantigens) or, alternatively, fail to present regulatory molecules that would normally prevent attack from the innate immune system;

- competent immune effector cells;

- a permissive tumour microenvironment allowing immune effector and helper cells effective access to the tumour sites.

Tests that identify whether these elements are present – or can be restored – in an individual patient may establish whether immuno-oncological therapy is feasible and rationally guide a personalized choice of treatment. In recent years a number of techniques have emerged that attempt to achieve this.

Establishing the presence of immune targets

Genomic instability is a hallmark of cancer; certain tumours, particularly those caused by prolonged exposure to DNA-damaging environmental factors or with impaired DNA repair capability such as cutaneous melanoma or smoking-induced lung cancer, carry a very high number of mutations and would be expected to present a large number of potentially immunogenic neoantigens.[1] These tumour types were identified early as promising targets for immuno-oncological agents and have proven in most cases to have significantly higher response rates to programmed cell death protein 1 (PD-1) axis blockade compared with less genetically damaged tumours such as uveal melanoma.[2]

The advent of affordable DNA sequencing platforms has allowed the assessment of mutational load in individual patient tumours. Tumour mutational burden is a measure of the number of mutations in a tumour genome, defined as the total number of mutations per coding area of a tumour genome. There is now unequivocal evidence that in multiple tumour types a high mutational burden is linked to enhanced response rates to immune checkpoint blockade; however, positive outcomes are also seen, although at lower frequencies, in less mutated tumours. The use of tumour mutational burden as a biomarker in the clinical setting is not widespread. In part this is due to the high cost and bioinformatics required to determine tumour mutational burden by whole exome sequencing. Mutational load of the genome may, however, be inferred from sequencing a smaller panel of a few hundred genes, which has led to the approval of some commercially available platforms such as FoundationOne (www.foundationmedicine.com) to aid clinical decision making. Tumour mutational burden has already begun to be measured in clinical practice: ipilimumab and nivolumab have recently been approved by the US Food and Drug Administration (FDA) for first line treatment of patients with advanced non-small-cell lung carcinoma (NSCLC) with ≥10 mutations per megabase.[3]

The relatively low negative predictive value of a high tumour mutational burden is likely due its statistical nature: tumours with few (or even a single) highly expressed or very strongly immunogenic neoantigens may be able to trigger just as strong an immune response as those with a high overall mutational burden. Extensive neoantigen presentation may also occur without concomitantly large-scale genetic changes: aberrant expression of normally suppressed protein fragments via changed splicing patterns, translation/transcription of alternative/cryptic reading frames, post-translational modifications and altered loading on to major histocompatibility complex (MHC) molecules may all be driven by mutations in a few critical genes in the respective pathways.

A high tumour mutational burden is associated with mutations in DNA polymerases, genes for DNA mismatch repair pathways or other changes resulting in microsatellite instability. In 2017, pembrolizumab was approved by the FDA for the treatment of patients with unresectable or metastatic solid tumours with high microsatellite instability or mismatch repair deficiency, becoming the first cancer treatment to be approved on the basis of a common biomarker rather than on the site of origin of the cancer.

Unsurprisingly, the MHC repertoire itself also plays a critical role.[4] Studies have shown that patients heterozygous for class I haplotypes have better outcomes, and that particular haplotypes may also be associated with differential response rates. Conversely, MHC class I downregulation is associated with lower levels of PD-1/ programmed death-ligand 1 (PD-L1) expression in several tumour types and has been identified as a potential resistance mechanism in patients receiving immune checkpoint inhibitors.

Establishing the presence of immune effector cells

In several cancers a clear link exists between absolute numbers of immune cells in the tumour microenvironment and outcomes.[5] Patients with tumours poor in immune cell infiltrates ('immune cold') have been shown to stand a lower chance of benefiting from anti-PD-1 therapies; the converse is true in patients with infiltrate-rich ('immune hot') tumours. This association is specific to the tumour type, with different cell populations more important in different contexts, although cluster of differentiation (CD) 8+, and to a lesser extent CD4+, T cells seem to stand out. Approximately one in three tumours are thought to have an inflamed tumour microenvironment (hot tumour inflammation signature or 'inflamed'), suggesting a pre-existing adaptive immune response; agents that cause reversal of local inhibitory factors (e.g. PD-1 and PD-L1 inhibitors) may be clinically successful in this group. Conversely, non-inflamed tumours (cold tumour inflammation signature or 'excluded' and 'desert') have low T cell infiltrates, which could suggest a failure of T cell trafficking or lack of activation of the host's immune system. Therapeutic approaches in these cases may be best focused on reversing these issues, e.g. with antiangiogenic agents or vaccines.

Currently, there are no regulatory approved assays to measure tumour inflammation, but a number are in development. Scoring systems have been proposed that include factors such as absolute and relative numbers of multiple immune cell types, location of cells (tumour centre vs periphery) and tumour expression of particular molecules of interest (MHC class I). Several have been validated in specific contexts and there is an ongoing effort to extend them using modern techniques. For example, the Immunoscore scoring system is based on the measurement of the density of two lymphocyte populations (CD3+ and CD8+ T cells) both in the core and in the invasive margin of the tumour in paraffin-embedded tissue and has been shown to provide a reliable estimate of the risk of recurrence in colorectal cancer.[6] Significant research activity in this area continues.

Determining the immune permissiveness of the tumour microenvironment

Identification of the presence of specific immune escape mechanisms in the tumour micro-environment is a promising predictive biomarker for the activity of immuno-oncological agents designed to counteract them; for example, PD-L1 expression has been validated as a predictive marker for the efficacy of pembrolizumab (an anti-PD-1 antibody) in NSCLC. Attempts to extend the success of this approach to other tumour types have resulted in poor positive and negative predictive values. A number of practical issues including lack of reproducibility across studies and multiple competing platforms – with arbitrary scoring systems and cut-offs – are partly responsible and are explored elsewhere in this book.

A larger issue is the concurrent presence of multiple tumour evasion mechanisms that vary across tumour types; synchronous assessment of multiple immunomodulatory pathways is necessary to allow sensible predictions about the activity of a given immuno-oncological agent in this context. Several studies have confirmed that specific transcription patterns correlate with outcomes, and based on this discovery gene expression arrays are currently in development as potential biomarkers.[7]

Establishing additional host factors

A number of host factors also contribute to the outcome of immunotherapy in a given individual; genetic (MHC haplotypes, polymorphisms in immune peptide-processing apparatus, T cell receptor [TCR] repertoire), nutritional, environmental (microbiome, previous exposure to viral antigens) and age-related changes have all been posited to play a role. There is significant evidence that single nucleotide polymorphisms (SNPs) play a major role in modulating both levels of immunity and the immune response and may play a role in development and activation of T cells. Detection of specific SNPs in the host may determine the response to or requirement for certain immunotherapy treatments. Other genetic variants including those seen in MHC genes as well as in genes encoding cytokines or associated with cytokine secretion may also play a role in the ability of the host to mount a successful immune response to tumour. There is also great interest in the role of the patient's microbiome in determining both response to immunotherapies and susceptibility to toxicities.[8] Interesting early data from preclinical mouse models suggest that manipulation of the gut microbiome may influence response to immunotherapy and there are many ongoing studies in this area to see whether this will translate to clinically relevant interventions.

Future prospects

The development of affordable genomic sequencing techniques, high-dimensional flow cytometry and improved bioinformatics capabilities is rapidly pushing the field forward. Machine learning-derived predictive algorithms allow affordable estimation of an individual patient's tumour mutational burden by extrapolating from sequencing a limited set of carefully selected genes.

Lessons learnt from in-depth analysis of the tumour microenvironment should allow the development and validation of tests that provide qualitatively comparable information via non-invasive/peripheral blood sampling means and that may be routinely employed in the clinic.

In the research setting, high-dimensional multiplex analysis of pure cell subpopulations from the tumour microenvironment is now achievable and can be downscaled to the single cell level. Synchronous evaluation of multiple cell types at the genomic, transcriptomic and proteomic level can provide highly personalized immune profiling. Probing of the immune peptidome of a given tumour and matching it to the host TCR repertoire will soon be within reach of investigators.

Advanced bioinformatics will facilitate the integration of high-dimensional '-omic' information into comprehensible scoring schemes that classify cancers according to modes of immune attack and escape, and eventually identify optimal treatment strategies bringing immuno-oncology to the precision medicine era.

References

1   Alexandrov LB, Nik-Zainal S, Wedge DC, *et al.* Signatures of mutational processes in human cancer. *Nature* 2013; 500: 415–21.

2   Yarchoan M, Hopkins A, Jaffee EM. Tumor mutational burden and response rate to PD-1 inhibition. *N Engl J Med* 2017; 377: 2500–1.

3   Hellmann MD, Ciuleanu TE, Pluzansk A, *et al.* Nivolumab plus ipilimumab in lung cancer with a high tumor mutational burden. *N Engl J Med* 2018; 378: 2093–104.

4   Chowell D, Morris LGT, Grigg CM, *et al.* Patient HLA class I genotype influences cancer response to checkpoint blockade immunotherapy. *Science* 2018; 359: 582–7.

5   Ganesan A-P, Clarke J, Wood O, *et al.* Tissue-resident memory features are linked to the magnitude of cytotoxic T cell responses in human lung cancer. *Nat Immunol* 2017; 18: 940–50.

6   Galon J, Mlecnik B, Bindea G, *et al.* Towards the introduction of the 'Immunoscore' in the classification of malignant tumours. *J Pathol* 2014; 232: 199–209.

7   Gnjatic S, Bronte V, Brunet LR, *et al.* Identifying baseline immune-related biomarkers to predict clinical outcome of immunotherapy. *J Immunother Cancer* 2017; 5: 44.

8   Zitvogel L, Ma Y, Raoult D, *et al.* The microbiome in cancer immunotherapy: diagnostic tools and therapeutic strategies. *Science* 2018; 359: 1366–70.

06 Difficulties in Assessment of PD-L1 Expression

John Gosney, Alexander Haragan

Introduction

Increased expression of programmed death-ligand 1 (PD-L1) is one mechanism neoplastic cells employ to protect themselves from immune attack. Binding of PD-L1 to its receptor, programmed cell death protein 1 (PD-1), results in inhibition of immune cells that would otherwise attack and destroy the tumour cell. Immunomodulatory drugs include immune checkpoint inhibitors that act on the PD-1/PD-L1 axis to interrupt this protective mechanism, thereby re-exposing the tumour to the immune system. These drugs have broadened and greatly improved treatment options for a variety of cancers, including non-small-cell lung carcinoma (NSCLC).[1–3] As might be expected, immunomodulatory drugs are generally more effective against tumours in which there is high expression of PD-L1 on either the tumour cells themselves or on tumour-infiltrating immune cells, hence the rationale for PD-L1 testing.[1,2,4,5]

Unfortunately, different immunochemical assays for detecting PD-L1 were developed for each immunomodulatory drug, resulting in a multitude of antibodies and platforms that were initially considered non-interchangeable. This, compounded by inherent heterogeneity of PD-L1 expression and the challenge of accurately quantifying its expression in tissue sections, has created a difficult environment for PD-L1 testing.[1,5,6]

Range of tests

Four anti-PD-1/anti-PD-L1 immunomodulatory drugs are currently licensed for the treatment of cancer: nivolumab, pembrolizumab, atezolizumab and avelumab. Further agents, including durvalumab, are in clinical trials but are currently unlicensed. During their clinical trials, each agent was developed with a different PD-L1 test. As shown in Table 6.1, not only do these agents employ different antibody clones but they are run on different platforms and have different cut-offs for determination of positivity.[1,4,6,7]

Inherent properties of PD-L1 expression

PD-L1 expression within a primary cancer, and between a primary tumour and its metastases, may be markedly heterogeneous, altering not only with time as the tumour evolves, but also spatially within the tumour.[6,7] Even across a small area of a tissue section, some tumour cells might demonstrate very strong expression and others very weak or no expression (Figure 6.1). Decisions to recommend treatment are based on a percentage score, usually in a small biopsy specimen, of PD-L1-positive tumour cells known as the tumour proportion score. It is often, however, difficult or impossible to know how truly representative such an assessment actually is of the overall tumour mass.

Table 6.1 PD-L1 assessment in NSCLC: antibodies, platforms and interpretation.

Anti–PD-L1 antibody	Immunomodulatory drug		
	Atezolizumab	Nivolumab, pembrolizumab, durvalumab[a]	Avelumab
Test	Ventana SP142	Dako 28-8, Dako 22C3, Ventana SP263	Dako 73-10
Platform	Ventana	Dako or Ventana	Dako
Interpretation	Tumour cells and immune cells	Tumour cells	Tumour cells
TPS cut-off	Tumour cells 0–3 (<1, 1–4, 5–49, ≥50) Immune cells 0–3 (<1, 1–4, 5–9, ≥10)	≥1%, ≥25%, ≥50% depending on drug and indication	≥1% in clinical trials

[a]Harmonization studies reveal close concordance between these three tests.[4,6,7]

TPS, tumour proportion score.

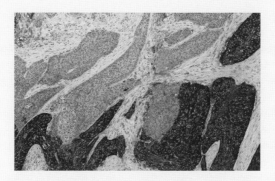

Figure 6.1 Expression of PD-L1 by a squamous cell carcinoma identified by immunochemistry using the Dako 22C3 antibody. There is striking heterogeneity of expression, which is strong and uniform in the right of the field and absent in the left. The scattered aggregates of small PD-L1-positive cells in the left of the field are infiltrating immune cells.

The use of cytology specimens, largely obtained from endoscopic bronchial ultrasound-guided aspirates, is even more problematic.[1] Not only were such specimens not used in clinical trials but also, more importantly, this cytology material is usually preserved in alcohol-based fixatives, which might reduce the antigenicity of PD-L1.[1,5]

Problems of interpretation

A further pragmatic and important difficulty lies in the rising demand for PD-L1 testing and the subsequent burden this places on individual pathologists and pathology services across the UK. Interpreting a PD-L1 test is not straightforward and may be challenging even to an experienced pathologist.[1,5,6]

Recent developments

Harmonization of tests

Considerable efforts have been made to harmonize PD-L1 tests (Table 6.1). Current evidence indicates that three clones, Dako 28–8, Dako 22C3 and Ventana SP263, are broadly equivalent, with the latter probably having the highest sensitivity.[4,6,7] As such, this test, originally developed as a companion diagnostic to durvalumab, has been given the European Conformity mark of approval to guide its use in patients being considered for pembrolizumab or nivolumab treatment.

The Ventana SP142 test appears to be less sensitive for detecting PD-L1 expression by tumour cells but more sensitive for detecting it on immune cells, hence the greater complexity of its assessment.[4,6,7] Conversely, the Dako 73–10 test appears to be more sensitive than the others. In practical terms, it is difficult to see how these two 'outliers' might be harmonized with those that are broadly similar in their sensitivity and specificity.

Heterogeneity

The implications of heterogeneity of PD-L1 expression within a tumour and between the tumour and its metastases are widely acknowledged. Attempts to assess heterogeneity and its clinical relevance have produced mixed results.[1,5,6] Unfortunately, these studies vary widely in their design and approach; have used different, sometimes 'research' anti-PD-L1 antibodies; and have often involved only a small number of samples. The few studies so far addressing concordance between histology and cytology specimens have shown encouraging results, suggesting that the problems with the latter are perhaps exaggerated and arise from inappropriate fixation and handling rather than from the quality of the specimen itself.[1]

Training and quality assurance

Technical quality of PD-L1 testing should be ensured by engagement of the laboratory in an appropriate external quality assurance scheme such as that run by Cancer Diagnostic Quality Assurance Services. Pathologists reporting PD-L1 tests should be familiar with the tumour type and, in the case of NSCLC, for example, ideally handle a minimum of 200 specimens annually. In addition, they should be a member of an external quality assurance scheme, such as that run in the UK under the auspices of the Association of Pulmonary Pathologists, and must have undergone the necessary training and certification.[1,6]

Alternative biomarkers and new therapeutics

Expression of PD-L1 is a fragile biomarker and work is underway to identify others to complement or maybe even replace it as a guide to the use of immunomodulatory drugs. Other potential biomarkers cover a broad range of targets and include tumour mutational burden, tumour acidity, interferon-γ activity, and various measurements of genetic variation and translational factors.[8-10]

It is likely that multiple biomarkers will eventually become validated for use alongside PD-L1 expression, and their combined interpretation and integration will be crucial. At present, however, there is still much to be done in developing such candidate biomarkers into tools that can be practically integrated into day-to-day practice.

Conclusion

 PD-L1 expression is by no means the perfect biomarker. The biological heterogeneity and multiplicity of antibodies and platforms, as well as difficulties in its interpretation, are serious drawbacks. Broadly speaking, however, it works; its relationship to the sensitivity of a tumour to immunomodulatory drugs is not in doubt and immunochemical assays have the advantages of being quick and cheap to perform.[1,3,5,6]

The applicability of small tissue and cytology specimens remains uncertain; however, evidence is mounting that these are suitable substrates, providing handling and fixation are appropriate and material is not wasted by unnecessary testing during initial diagnosis and tumour typing.

In the future it is likely that PD-L1 immunochemical expression will be complemented, if not replaced, by other assessments of tumour immune biology, the 'cancer immunogram' being an example.[9,10] For the moment, however, assessing PD-L1 expression by immunochemical assay is the only validated means of guiding the use of immunomodulatory drugs in cancer and it is essential that it is done well.

References

1   Cree I, Booton R, Cane P, *et al*. PD-L1 testing for lung cancer in the UK: recognizing the challenges for implementation. *Histopathology* 2016; 69: 177–86.

2   Takada K, Toyokawa G, Shoji F, *et al*. The significance of the PD-L1 expression in non-small-cell lung cancer: trenchant double swords as predictive and prognostic markers. *Clin Lung Cancer* 2017; 19: 120–9.

3   Khunger M, Jain P, Rakshit S, *et al*. Safety and efficacy of PD-1/PD-L1 inhibitors in treatment-naive and chemotherapy-refractory patients with non-small-cell lung cancer: a systematic review and meta-analysis. *Clin Lung Cancer* 2018; 19: e335–48.

4   Ratcliffe MJ, Sharpe A, Midha A, *et al*. Agreement between programmed cell death ligand-1 diagnostic assays across multiple protein expression cutoffs in non-small cell lung cancer. *Clin Cancer Res* 2017; 23: 3585–91.

5   Ilie M, Hofman V, Dietel M, *et al*. Assessment of the PD-L1 status by immunohistochemistry: challenges and perspectives for therapeutic strategies in lung cancer patients. *Virchows Arch* 2016; 468: 511–25.

6   Büttner R, Gosney J, Skov B, *et al*. Programmed death-ligand 1 immunohistochemistry testing: a review of analytical assays and clinical implementation in non-small-cell lung cancer. *J Clin Oncol* 2017; 35: 3867–76.

7   Hirsch F, McElhinny A, Stanforth D, *et al*. PD-L1 immunohistochemistry assays for lung cancer: results from phase 1 of the blueprint PD-L1 IHC assay comparison project. *J Thorac Oncol* 2017; 12: 208–22.

8   Gnjatic S, Bronte V, Brunet LR, *et al*. Identifying baseline immune-related biomarkers to predict clinical outcome of immunotherapy. *J Immunother Cancer* 2017; 5: 44.

9   Chen D, Mellman I. Elements of cancer immunity and the cancer-immune set point. *Nature* 2017; 541: 321–30.

10 Blank CU, Haanen JB, Ribas A, Schumacher TN. Cancer immunology. The 'cancer immunogram'. *Science* 2016; 352: 658–60.

07 Radiological Assessment of Immunotherapy

Beth Shepherd

Introduction

Cancer immunotherapy is presenting new challenges in the imaging evaluation of treatment response and the diagnosis of treatment-related complications. Accurate and reproducible assessment of response requires familiarization with the emerging patterns following immunotherapy. The underlying mechanisms of immunotherapy expose the patient to the risk of immune-related adverse events (irAEs). Timely and comprehensive assessment of irAEs is important for prompt and appropriate clinical management.

Assessment of disease response

Assessment of disease response following immunotherapy requires specific knowledge for accurate radiological interpretation.

- Treatment response may be associated with a significant delay in the decrease of the tumour burden. This delay is attributable to the time interval required for the immune system to mount the desired response through activation and expansion of effector cell populations.

- Clinically significant stabilization of disease describes a tumour burden that may remain static for a prolonged period after treatment and may or may not eventually demonstrate a decrease in volume. This is thought to be more significant in terms of responses to immunotherapy compared with similar findings following conventional cytotoxic therapy.

- Pseudo-progression, or flare effect, may herald a delayed response to treatment after an initial increase in tumour volume. It occurs immediately after treatment within the so-called flare time window and may be a transient increase in tumour size or the emergence of 'new' metastases due to immune cell infiltration of existing deposits, with or without significant associated oedema. Current thinking suggests this phenomenon is over-reported. It is more likely that apparent pseudo-progression, be it of existing disease or emerging metastases, reflects true tumour growth in the lag time before the effective immune response.

These patterns of response are reflected in the recommended radiological surveillance following treatment with immunotherapy. Imaging assessment after completion of treatment should be made with two consecutive follow-up studies performed at least 4 weeks apart, mainly to negate the effect of a delayed response. If new or enlarging disease is observed immediately after the completion of treatment, repeat imaging should be undertaken at least 4 weeks later to assess further changes. This addresses the potential confusion of pseudo-progression.

It is important to be able to assess treatment response both accurately and reproducibly. For conventional cytotoxic agents the Response Evaluation Criteria in Solid Tumors (RECIST) (version 1.1) are currently used. These have their own inherent shortcomings but significantly so in the context of immunotherapy. To reflect the differences between traditional RECIST and the concepts discussed above, specific immune-based response criteria (iRECIST) have been published.

The most recent uses unidimensional measurements to provide a standardized approach to treatment response.[1]

Future developments in the assessment of treatment response will not only include the refinement of these criteria but also a change in the way tumour burden is measured. At present we use anatomically measurable disease to assess treatment efficacy. Simple measurements of tumour burden do not take into consideration changeable cellular, functional or metabolic data from disease sites, such as MR diffusion-weighted imaging or fluorodeoxyglucose (FDG) avidity. These alterations may precede standard measurable changes in disease volume and in some cases may be the only indicator of disease response. The use of MR diffusion-weighted imaging may give important information about changes in tumour cellularity after treatment.[2] An early prediction of treatment response is extremely advantageous; following immunotherapy, one of the main hurdles is differentiating the required inflammatory response from genuine tumour proliferation. To help address this issue, novel PET radiotracers are being developed that aim to distinguish between cellular proliferation and cell death.[3] It is envisaged that routine assessment of morphological, metabolic, cellular and functional parameters will become the norm.

irAEs

The use of immunotherapeutic agents is associated with a wide spectrum of irAEs reflecting the underlying mechanisms of immunotherapy. This is due to the induction of autoimmunity and the propagation of a proinflammatory state. The breadth and potential severity of these complications are becoming better appreciated in the clinical setting. Adverse effects involve multiple organs including gastrointestinal, renal, hepatic, cardiac, neurological, pulmonary, skin, muscular, endocrine and haematological systems. irAEs may occur after the first treatment, but most commonly several weeks later, with the majority of irAEs occurring within the treatment induction period. Some irAEs, however, may have a significant delay and occur well beyond the cessation of treatment. There is thought to be a positive correlation between tumour response and irAE risk, which is easy to envisage given the biological mechanisms of treatment.

There may be significant preventable morbidity, or even mortality, if irAEs are misdiagnosed and consequently not optimally managed. An irAE may be incorrectly diagnosed as an unrelated entity, which may lead to inappropriate treatment, a delay in correct management and a risk of further complications. Features of irAEs may also be mistaken for treatment failure or metastatic disease progression, which may result in the unnecessary termination of potentially effective treatment.

One of most problematic features is that almost all of the radiological manifestations are non-specific, in that they may be attributed to a number of other aetiologies, which makes diagnosis more challenging. Often patients are treated concurrently for other problems such as infection. The diagnosis of an irAE is sometimes a diagnosis of exclusion and is often made more definitively once there has been a positive response to the steroid treatment

Radiological abnormalities potentially attributable to immunotherapy may be clinically evident or clinically silent. More frequent clinically evident irAEs include colitis and hypophysitis. A common clinically silent irAE is sarcoid-like lymphadenopathy, but this group also includes diffuse retroperitoneal stranding.

- Colitis is an important complication that requires prompt diagnosis and treatment. It is associated with the highest mortality of all irAEs, usually as a result of a delay between presentation and the correct diagnosis and management. Colitis in this context has been described in two separate patterns. The first is diffuse colitis, which may be seen on a plain abdominal film with bowel wall thickening and thumbprinting. Generally it is diagnosed on CT, with features including concentric mural thickening, mucosal hyperenhancement, pericolic inflammatory stranding and an injected mesentery (Figure 7.1). Complications of colitis may also

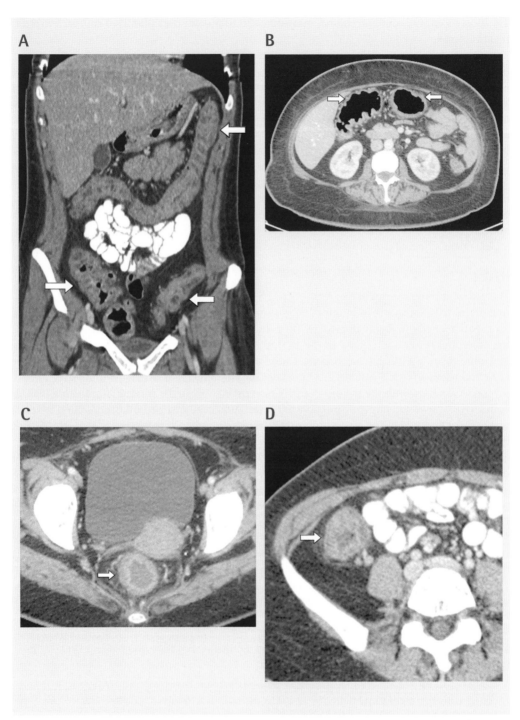

Figure 7.1 Diffuse colitis shown on post-contrast CT. (A) Extensive mural thickening of the entire colon (normally the bowel wall should be as thin as a pencil line). The bowel wall thickening is of low density in keeping with oedema. (B) Prominent or 'injected' vessels in the colonic mesentery. (C) Concentric mural thickening of the rectum, demonstrating proctitis. (D) Mural thickening of the ascending colon with adjacent inflammatory stranding and enlarged lymph nodes.

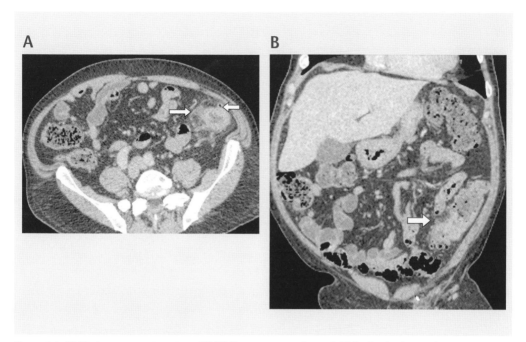

Figure 7.2 SCAD shown on post-contrast CT. (A) Short segment of mural thickening in the proximal sigmoid colon with underlying diverticulosis (small arrow); marked associated inflammatory stranding. (B) Same findings in the coronal plane.

be observed, including perforation. The second pattern is of segmental colitis associated with diverticulosis (SCAD). The distinction is not just academic, as SCAD usually requires antibiotic as well as steroid treatment (Figure 7.2).

- Other abdominal manifestations include hepatitis, which may present clinically or as an incidental finding. Hepatitis is most commonly seen on CT with periportal oedema and hypo-attenuation of the liver secondary to oedema. Pancreatitis is a rare complication but may be seen on CT or MRI as an engorged 'sausage-like' gland.

- Endocrinopathies include hypophysitis and thyroiditis, both readily identifiable on imaging. Hypophysitis may be identified on multiple imaging modalities including CT, where an enhancing soft tissue mass involves the pituitary. MRI shows enlargement of the pituitary gland with, usually, homogenous enhancement and a thickened infundibulum (Figure 7.3). PET-CT can demonstrate increased FDG avidity within the sella. It is important that it is not mistaken for metastatic disease. Thyroiditis is usually demonstrated on ultrasound with hyporeflectivity, coarse texture and increased vascularity of the gland in the context of thyrotoxicosis.

- Immune-related arthritis is most often a clinical diagnosis but may be seen on several imaging modalities, including PET-CT, where there is increased FDG uptake within a joint, which is usually symmetrical and in multiple joints. Myositis is usually clinically silent but may be seen radiologically with increased enhancement or FDG avidity in muscle. Similar imaging features occur with neuropathies.

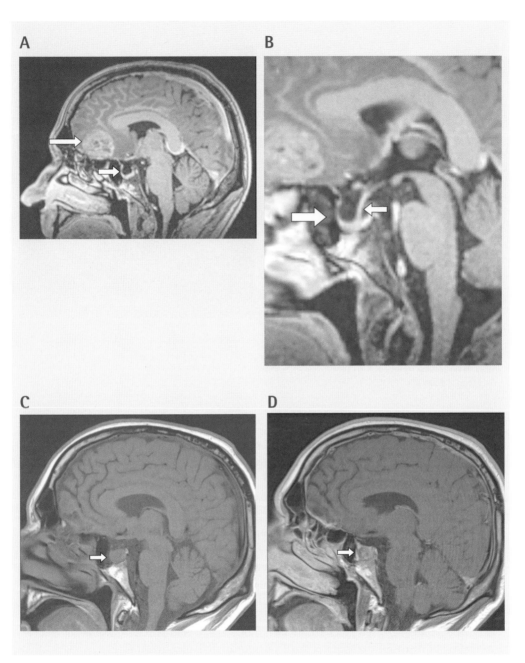

Figure 7.3 Hypophysitis. (A) Pretreatment MRI: post-contrast sagittal T1 shows a normal pituitary gland; the majority of the sella contains cerebrospinal fluid (little arrow). Note the frontal lobe metastasis from melanoma (big arrow). (B) Enlarged image as above showing normal structures in the pituitary fossa (big arrow), including a thin enhancing infundibulum (little arrow). (C) After frontal lobe metastasectomy and combination immunotherapy the patient presented with worsening headaches and it was feared there was metastatic recurrence. Sagittal T1 shows significant enlargement of the pituitary gland. (D) As above, following gadolinium contrast enhancement. The pituitary shows slightly patchy but fairly homogenous enhancement. No residual frontal mass is seen.

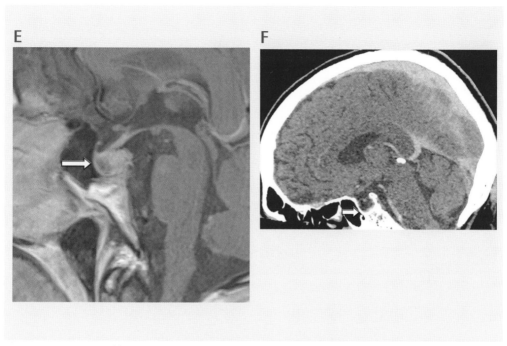

Figure 7.3 (Continued) (E) Enlarged image of above, showing thickening of the infundibulum. (F) Following treatment with steroids and an appropriate time interval, post-contrast CT with sagittal reformats shows the pituitary volume returned to normal.

- Thoracic manifestations are less common but include pneumonitis, myocarditis and pericarditis. Immune-related pneumonitis is a serious and potentially fatal condition. It may occur at a significant interval after treatment. Often plain chest X-ray is normal unless the process is very advanced. CT is usually used for diagnosis; the most common feature on CT is ground glass change which may be diffuse or patchy but usually symmetrical. There may be associated reticular opacities and nodular change; in more severe cases there may be dense consolidation (Figures 7.4–7.6). The main differential for pneumonitis in this setting is infection, potentially with atypical agents including fungal and *Pneumocystis* species. An often clinically silent thoracic manifestation is sarcoid-like lymphadenopathy (Figure 7.7). It is important not to mistake it for metastatic disease: sarcoid-like lymphadenopathy is normally symmetrical; fine needle aspiration or biopsy may help to differentiate the two if clinically required.

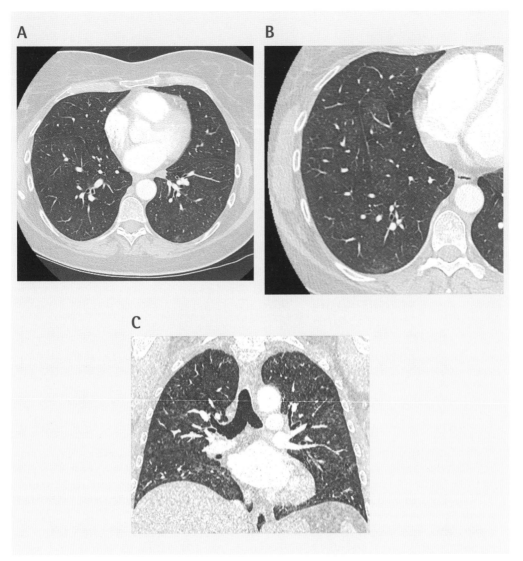

Figure 7.4 Pneumonitis shown on post-contrast CT in lung windows. (A) Minor patchy ground glass change: appearances may be very subtle and comparison with previous imaging is extremely useful. Early changes are often seen in retrospect on the original imaging. Radiologists should perhaps have a lower threshold for raising potential pneumonitis if the patient is known to have undergone immunotherapy. (B) Patchy ground glass change: more normal areas of lung appear darker. (C) Changes as above on coronal reformats.

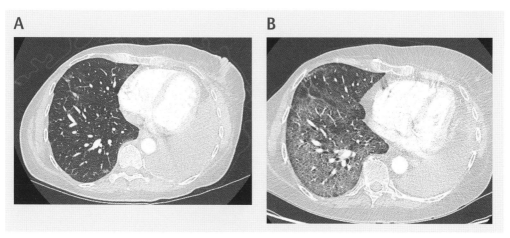

Figure 7.5 Pneumonitis shown on post-contrast CT in lung windows. (A) Left pneumonectomy with very minor ground glass and nodular change at the right base. (B) At an interval of several weeks the patient became more symptomatic and progressive changes were seen on imaging. As well as ground glass change and nodularity some reticular thickening is seen.

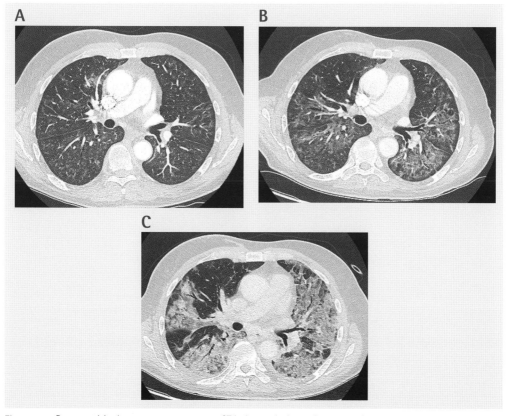

Figure 7.6 Pneumonitis shown on post-contrast CT in lung windows, demonstrating progressively worse imaging findings that correlated with the patient's symptomatology. (A) Subtle nodular and ground glass change in a fairly symmetrical distribution. (B) Demonstrating interval progression. (C) Symptomatic deterioration: further imaging showed progression of the pneumonitic changes with consolidation now evident.

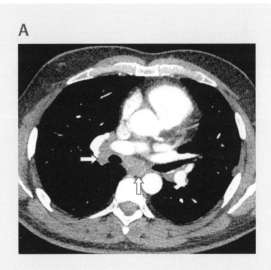

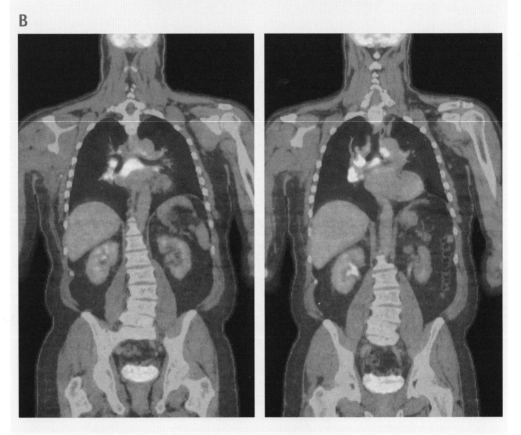

Figure 7.7 Sarcoid-like lymphadenopathy. (A) Post-contrast CT shows mediastinal and bihilar lymphadenopathy. (B) This lymphadenopathy demonstrated significant avidity on PET-CT. Fine needle aspiration of an FDG-avid supraclavicular node was performed in this patient to differentiate from metastatic disease.

Conclusion

- Accurate and reproducible radiological assessment of treatment response needs to take into account specific immunotherapy response patterns. These also guide the timing of follow-up imaging.
- There is an anticipated move away from response assessment relying on disease volume, with a move to reflect cellular, functional and metabolic changes.
- The timely and accurate assessment of irAEs is paramount for patient safety, particularly as novel agents are increasingly in routine clinical use.

References

1   Seymour L, Bogearts J, Perrone A, *et al*. iRECIST: guidelines for response criteria for use in trials testing immunotherapeutics. *Lancet Oncol* 2017; 18: e143–52.

2   Li SP, Padhani AR. Tumor response assessments with diffusion and perfusion MRI. *J Magn Reson Imaging* 2012; 35: 745–63.

3   Bauckneht M, Piva R, Sambuceti G, *et al*. Evaluation of response to immune checkpoint inhibitors: is there a role for positron emission tomography? *World J Radiol* 2017; 9: 27–33.

Further reading

- Chiou VL, Burotto M. Pseudoprogression and immune-related response in solid tumors. *J Clin Oncol* 2015; 33: 3541–3.

- Kwak J, Tirumani S, Van den Abbeele A, *et al*. Cancer immunotherapy: imaging assessment of novel treatment response patterns and immune-related adverse events. *Radiographics* 2015; 35: 424–37.

- Nishino M, Tirumani S, Ramaiya, N, Hodi F. Cancer immunotherapy and immune-related response assessment: the role of the radiologists in the new arena of cancer treatment. *Eur J Radiol* 2015; 84: 1259–68.

08 Combination Immunotherapies: Multimodality Treatment

Paul D. Nathan

Introduction

Immunotherapy with immune checkpoint inhibitors (ICPIs) delivers profound benefit to a subset of patients. Many patients, however, have disease that is unresponsive to current treatment from the outset (primary resistant disease) or have disease that relapses following a period of initial benefit (acquired resistance). Strategies to improve on single-agent ICPI activity include combining these drugs with other drugs of the same or a different class.

The principle of combining drugs in an attempt to overcome resistance underpins much of the development of modern chemotherapy. Combination regimens are frequently the standard of care for many tumours in both the curative and palliative settings. These regimens result from clinical trials in which the design compares a new combination against a historical single-agent treatment. Two drugs are frequently more active than a single agent using conventional efficacy criteria (response rate, progression-free survival [PFS] and overall survival [OS]); thus, the combination becomes the new standard of care.

Trials rarely examine whether combination therapy confers greater benefit than sequential treatment with all components of the combination. As combination therapy may be associated with increased toxicity, this is an important but usually unanswered question. Once a combination has become a standard of care it may be difficult to perform a study in which patients are randomized to receive combination components given sequentially, owing to an ethical concern that they risk receiving a less effective treatment. The ideal time to test whether a combination is superior to sequenced treatment is therefore before the combination has become a standard of care; however, it may not be in a sponsor's interest to perform such a study. Detection of a synergistic rather than an additive signal would give confidence that patients derive significant benefit from combination treatment.

Combinations of ICPIs

Combination programmed cell death protein 1 (PD-1) and cytotoxic T lymphocyte-associated protein 4 (CTLA-4) inhibition has become a standard of care in both melanoma and renal cell carcinoma (RCC), delivering significant benefit over single-agent ICPI therapy in both diseases. In melanoma, ipilimumab in combination with nivolumab showed superior efficacy over single-agent nivolumab or ipilimumab.[1] At 36 months' minimum follow-up, median OS was 37.6 months in the nivolumab group and 19.9 months in the ipilimumab group but had not been reached in the combination group. The HR for OS for combination ipilimumab plus nivolumab vs ipilimumab was 0.55 ($p<0.001$) and for single-agent nivolumab vs ipilimumab it was 0.65 ($p<0.001$). In RCC, combination ipilimumab plus nivolumab was compared with sunitinib, a standard of care tyrosine kinase inhibitor targeting the vascular endothelial growth factor (VEGF) receptor.[2] Ipilimumab plus nivolumab delivered an improvement in OS (HR 0.63; $p<0.001$). Combination immunotherapy also induced a significantly higher response rate compared with sunitinib (42% vs 27%, respectively) Combination ipilimumab and nivolumab in non-small-cell lung carcinoma (NSCLC) showed a highly significant improvement in PFS and response rate compared with chemotherapy or single-agent nivolumab in patients whose tumours contained a high mutational burden.[3] The benefit appeared to be independent of programmed death-ligand 1 (PD-L1) expression at a 1% immunohistochemistry cut-off: 1 year PFS was 42.6% with nivolumab plus ipilimumab vs 13.2% with chemotherapy; median PFS was 7.2 months vs 5.5 months, respectively (HR for disease progression or death, 0.58; 97.5% CI 0.41, 0.81; $p<0.001$).

The toxicity of combination CTLA-4 and PD-1 inhibition is significantly greater than that seen with a single-agent ICPI. The dose of ipilimumab appears to be the most significant driver of toxicity with this combination. In patients with advanced melanoma, ipilimumab (3 mg/kg) combined with nivolumab (1 mg/kg) for combination induction, every 3 weeks in four doses, and single-agent nivolumab (3 mg/kg every 2 weeks) for maintenance resulted in 39% of patients discontinuing treatment because of treatment-related toxicity and a 59% incidence of grades 3–4 adverse events.[1] This compares with treatment discontinuation rates of 7.7% in the nivolumab group and 14.8% in the ipilimumab group.[1] In patients with advanced RCC, ipilimumab (1 mg/kg) in combination with nivolumab (3 mg/kg), at the same schedule as the melanoma dose, resulted in only 22% of patients discontinuing treatment due to treatment-related adverse events.[2] Academic studies are exploring whether the dose of ipilimumab may be further reduced. The PRISM study (EudraCT 2017–001476–33) will randomize patients between the standard RCC dose of ipilimumab plus nivolumab and a reduced ipilimumab schedule where ipilimumab is given once every 3 months.

Agents that target a number of other immune checkpoints are in advanced stages of development. These are described in Chapter 2 and are most frequently being tested in combination with PD-1 or PD-L1 ICPIs.

Combinations with targeted therapies

A number of targeted treatments are standards of care in many diseases and are being assessed in combination with ICPIs. These include serine/threonine-protein kinase B-Raf (BRAF) and mitogen-activated protein kinase kinase (MEK) inhibitors in melanoma, VEGF receptor inhibitors in RCC, and epidermal growth factor (EGF) receptor inhibitors in lung and head and neck cancers. There is preclinical evidence that the tumour microenvironment can change upon exposure to a targeted agent, inducing not only tumour cell death but also the generation of a reactive infiltration of lymphocytes. The concept of combining ICPIs with targeted agents is therefore an attempt to expand and further activate the tumour-infiltrating lymphocyte population induced by treatment with the targeted agent.

The most advanced studies are currently in melanoma and RCC. Vemurafenib, a BRAF inhibitor, was found to induce hepatotoxicity in combination with ipilimumab in a phase I study[4] and was also found to be problematic in combination with nivolumab.[5] Similarly, a phase I study of the EGF receptor inhibitor osimertinib in combination with the anti-PD-L1 antibody durvalumab was stopped because of an increased incidence of interstitial lung disease.[6] By contrast, vemurafenib in combination with cobimetinib and atezolizumab does appear to be better tolerated.[7] Dabrafenib (a BRAF inhibitor) plus trametinib (a MEK inhibitor) are in a phase III study (ClinicalTrials.gov NCT02967692) in combination with spartalizumab (PDR001, a PD-1 inhibitor).

In RCC, three combinations of anti-PD-1 or anti-PD-L1 antibodies plus VEGF-targeted agents are currently in phase III clinical trials: avelumab with axitinib (ClinicalTrials.gov NCT02493751), atezolizumab with bevacizumab (ClinicalTrials.gov NCT02420821) and pembrolizumab with cabozantinib (ClinicalTrials.gov NCT03149822).

Combinations with other classes of immunotherapy

IDO inhibitors block the activity of indoleamine 2,3-dioxygenase, which metabolizes the essential amino acid tryptophan. Tryptophan depletion results in T cell suppression and is an important pathway in avoiding placental rejection. IDO activity in the tumour microenvironment is thought to suppress T cell activation and immune-mediated anticancer response. Encouraging activity of IDO inhibitors in combination with ICPIs in early phase clinical trials has led to a number of phase III studies in melanoma, RCC, lung, bladder, and head and neck cancers. Early reports from a phase III study of epacadostat in combination with pembrolizumab in melanoma have, however, been negative;[8] more clinical data from this combination are awaited.

Many other immunotherapeutic interventions are being investigated in combination with ICPIs. These include viral therapies, vaccines and the bi-specific molecule IMCgp100, which links an engineered T cell receptor specific for a gp100 peptide expressed on many melanomas to an anti-cluster of differentiation (CD) 3 moiety which binds to and activates T cells.

Combination with chemotherapy

Pembrolizumab in combination with chemotherapy in NSCLC was recently shown to very significantly improve 1 year OS from 49.4% to 69.2% (HR 0.49; $p<0.001$).[9] It will be interesting to discover whether chemotherapy can help potentiate immune responses to ICPIs in other clinical settings. Not only would this have implications for diseases in which chemotherapy remains the backbone of systemic treatment it would also raise the possibility that ICPI and chemotherapy combinations may have a role in malignancies for which chemotherapy has little current place.

Combination with radiotherapy

The abscopal effect refers to an improvement in distant disease following a local treatment and has most frequently been described after treatment of a tumour deposit with radiotherapy. Multiple clinical cases have been reported in a variety of cancers. Preclinical data demonstrate enhancement of immune responses with fractionated high-dose radiotherapy, which appears to result in immunogenic cell death.[10] Clinical outcomes for patients receiving radiotherapy before or concomitantly with ICPIs appear better;[11] however, larger prospective studies are needed to further investigate this finding.

A number of clinical trials are underway which examine differing fractionation regimens in combination with immunotherapy. Unfortunately the PERM trial,[12] which prospectively attempted to randomize radiotherapy (24 Gy in three fractions) in melanoma patients receiving pembrolizumab and therefore measure the size of the abscopal effect, has closed due to poor accrual. Further work is required in this area.

Conclusion

 ICPIs targeting PD-1 or PD-L1 have become a standard of care in a number of cancers. Many patients experience significant benefit; however, a majority of patients do not. There is therefore a clinical need to build on this advance; combining these agents with others of the same or a different class is an obvious way forward. It is likely that a number of the combinations described in this chapter will become new standards of care over the next few years. Academic studies with robust translational science will be required to assess whether combinations confer a significant advantage over single agents used sequentially.

References

1 Wolchok J, Chiarion-Sileni V, González R, *et al.* Overall survival with combined nivolumab and ipilimumab in advanced melanoma. *N Engl J Med* 2017; 377: 1345–56.

2 Motzer RJ, Tannir NM, McDermott DF, *et al.* Nivolumab plus ipilimumab versus sunitinib in advanced renal-cell carcinoma. *N Engl J Med* 2018; 378: 1277–90.

3 Hellmann MD, Ciuleanu TE, Pluzanski A, *et al.* Nivolumab plus ipilimumab in lung cancer with a high tumor mutational burden. *N Engl J Med* 2018; 378: 2093–104.

4 Ribas A, Hodi FS, Callahan M, *et al.* Hepatotoxicity with combination of vemurafenib and ipilimumab. *N Engl J Med* 2013; 368: 1365–6.

5 Arenbergerova M, Mrazova I, Horazdovsky J, *et al.* Toxic epidermal necrolysis induced by vemurafenib after nivolumab failure. *J Eur Acad Dermatol Venereol* 2017; 31: e253–4.

6 Ahn MJ, Yang J, Yu H, *et al.* 136O: Osimertinib combined with durvalumab in *EGFR*-mutant non-small cell lung cancer: results from the TATTON phase Ib trial. *J Thorac Oncol* 2016; 11 (4 suppl): S115.

7 Sullivan RJ, González R, Lewis KD, *et al.* Atezolizumab (A) + cobimetinib (C) + vemurafenib (V) in *BRAF*V600-mutant metastatic melanoma (mel): updated safety and clinical activity. *J Clin Oncol* 2017; 35 (suppl): abstract 3063.

8 Long G, Dummer R, Hamid O, *et al.* Epacadostat (E) plus pembrolizumab (P) versus pembrolizumab alone in patients (pts) with unresectable or metastatic melanoma: results of the phase 3 ECHO-301/KEYNOTE-252 study. *J Clin Oncol* 2018; 36 (suppl): abstract 108.

9 Gandhi L, Rodríguez-Abreu D, Gadgeel S, *et al.* Pembrolizumab plus chemotherapy in metastatic non-small-cell lung cancer. *N Engl J Med* 2018; 378: 2078–92.

10 Dewan MZ, Galloway AE, Kawashima N, *et al.* Fractionated but not single-dose radiotherapy induces an immune-mediated abscopal effect when combined with anti-CTLA-4 antibody. *Clin Cancer Res* 2009; 15: 5379–88.

11 Escorcia FE, Postow MA, Barker CA. Radiotherapy and immune checkpoint blockade for melanoma: a promising combinatorial strategy in need of further investigation. *Cancer J* 2017; 23: 32–9.

12 Yip K, Melcher A, Harrington K, *et al.* Pembrolizumab in combination with radiotherapy for metastatic melanoma: introducing the PERM trial. *Clin Oncol (R Coll Radiol)* 2018; 30: 201–3.

09 Future Vaccine Strategies in Cancer Immunotherapy

Peter Selby, Adel Samson, Alan Melcher, Richard Vile

Introduction

The recent positive and exciting steps forward in the science and clinical applications of cancer immunotherapy are presented and discussed in this book. Progress in cancer immunotherapy has always depended critically on increasing knowledge of the underlying mechanisms of the immune response to cancer. Key areas of scientific understanding required to take cancer immunotherapy further forward, however, remain:

- What antigenic determinants may most effectively stimulate an anticancer immune response?

- What is the best biological context for antigen presentation to promote anticancer responses?

- What non-specific stimulation, or removal of inhibition, of the immune response, may be used to enhance clinical efficacy?

- How may we best combine vaccines and non-specific therapies?

Early attempts at non-specific enhancement of the immune response to cancer involved traditional adjuvants, often based on mycobacteria, or the systemic use of large doses of cytokines such as interleukin (IL)-2, IL-12 and IL-21. These are capable of enhancing immune responses to cancer in humans and do have some clinical efficacy but are poorly tolerated. More recently the use of immune checkpoint inhibitors (ICPIs) has non-specifically reduced inhibition of anticancer immune responses and has proved effective (covered elsewhere in this book). Even though they may also reduce inhibition of anti-self immune responses in some patients, they are more clinically tolerable when compared with the earlier strategies.

Tumour-associated antigens (TAAs) are found in both tumour and normal tissue but are over-expressed on tumour cells and/or expressed on dispensable tumour cells (e.g. cluster of differentiation [CD] 19 on B cell malignancies).[1] Examples of TAAs include human telomerase reverse transcriptase and survivin. On the other hand, tumour-specific antigens (TSAs) are expressed only in tumour cells. TSAs are usually either neoantigens, resulting from the products of somatic gene mutations, such as the abnormal protein of mutated *RAS*, or abnormally expressed cancer testis antigens such as melanoma-associated antigen (MAGE). Functionally, TAAs are more likely to be tolerated by the immune system due to their normal self-expression, whereas TSAs are, by definition, immunologically non-self.

Our knowledge of the presentation of antigenic determinants on cancer cells that will stimulate an immune response has advanced steadily (Figure 9.1). TAAs have been explored as the basis of cancer vaccines or specific adoptive cellular therapy with some success. Most notably, recently, targeting antigen expression on lymphoid cells through the adoptive transfer of chimeric antigen receptor cells specific to CD19 in refractory acute lymphoid leukaemia or relapsed B cell lymphoma was successful.[1] Some success has been reported using vaccines based on tumour lysates often mixed with antigen-presenting cells. In general, however, making use of TAAs that are present on

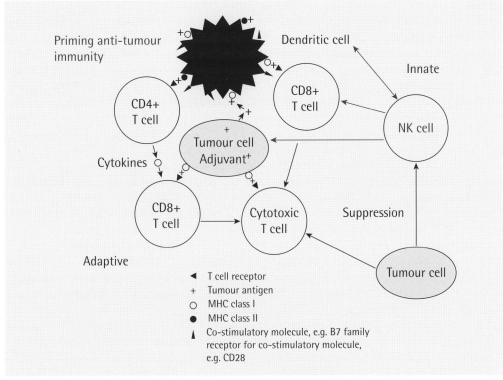

Figure 9.1 The immune response to cancer. The figure summarizes how tumour antigens are processed by dendritic cells and presented to CD4+ and CD8+ T cells in association with major histocompatibility complex (MHC) class I and class II. Co-stimulatory molecules and cytokines provide essential additional signals to stimulate an anticancer immune response. Innate immune responses may also mediate an anticancer effect through, for example, natural killer (NK) cells. The adaptive immune response is modulated by a range of suppressor mechanisms.

normal tissues or tumour lysates has not yet resulted in effective vaccines for most solid tumours. Even when TAAs are overexpressed on cancer cells, their expression on normal tissues may still limit selective anticancer efforts. The combination of TAAs as vaccines together with ICPIs is being explored in an attempt to enhance clinical efficacy.

Tumour neoantigens

Targeting TSAs may hold greater promise as the basis of effective cancer vaccines in the future, owing to their potential to elicit a highly selective anticancer immune response. The first immunogenic neoantigen was identified in Brussels by the Ludwig Institute for Cancer Research.[2] Prior to these experiments, the existence of neoantigens was implied by the generation of immunogenic variants in mouse tumour lines by treating non-immunogenic syngeneic mouse tumour cell transfers with chemical mutagens. The immunogenic variants are recognized by cytolytic T lymphocytes. The cloning of the gene for the P91 antigen represented a significant step forward.[2] This was followed by the identification of multiple neoepitopes on tumours as a result of mutagenesis. As genomic sequencing has advanced, we have been able to identify and predict the immunogenicity of neoantigens, with encouraging findings in mouse experiments.[2,3] Neoantigen formation and elimination play an important role in tumour biology. For instance, it is believed that the development of cancers may be eliminated at an early stage by a process called 'immunoediting', in which it is believed T cell recognition may be used to destroy developing cancers. Matsushita *et al.*[3] characterized the early neoantigens on mouse sarcomas and used prediction algorithms to identify potential rejection antigens. Outgrowing tumours lacked these antigens. Neoantigens are also important in tumour therapy. For instance, Castle *et al.*[4] sequenced B16 murine melanoma exomic DNA and showed it carried almost 1000 somatic point mutation neoantigens, half in expressed genes. Peptide vaccines based on these yielded tumour control.

Saini *et al.*[5] summarized the evidence. There is a consistent association between the presence of a high mutational load on tumours (generating neoantigens) and the probability of improved clinical outcomes for patients treated with ICPIs. They identified nine studies supporting the finding including a link between neoantigens due to mutagenesis and survival in melanoma patients treated with ICPIs. For example, Snyder *et al.*[6] showed clearly the association between neoepitope formation and benefit from ICPIs. When exomes from patients treated with cytotoxic T lymphocyte-associated protein 4 (CTLA-4) blockade were sequenced, mutational load was associated with the degree of clinical benefit. Furthermore, Snyder *et al.*[6] identified candidate tumour neoantigens for each patient associated with benefit in a group of patients, and had similar findings in a second separate, confirmatory, set of patients (Figure 9.2). The patterns of neoantigen formation in tumours seem to be quite tumour-specific and reflect the underlying biological processes of carcinogenesis in that tumour type. For example, lung and head and neck tumours show mutagenic patterns compatible with carcinogenesis from cigarette smoke; melanoma shows mutation

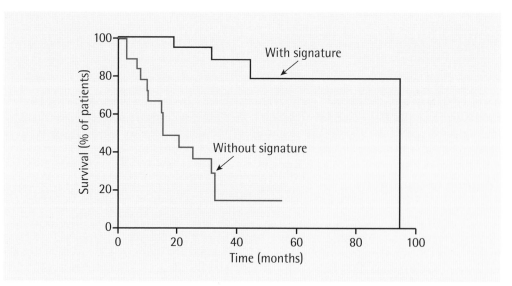

Figure 9.2 Survival of patients who expressed a neoepitope signature (*n*=20) compared with survival of patients without the signature (*n*=19) after treatment with ICPIs. A superior outcome was seen in patients expressing the neoepitope signature (*p*<0.001) (adapted from Snyder *et al.*[6]).

patterns linked to mutagenesis by ultraviolet light; many tumour types show patterns attributed to the apolipoprotein B mRNA-editing enzyme, catalytic polypeptide-like (APOBEC) family of cytokine deaminases.[7]

Personalized neoantigen vaccines

Insights into the importance of specific mutations forming neoantigens and their association with the immune response have led to initiatives to characterize the 'mutanome' of tumours as a tool for innovative vaccine development.[8] These studies use sophisticated structural biology and predictive algorithms to generate vaccines that are personalized for each patient. Preliminary results of this strategy are encouraging.[8] For example, Sahin et al.,[8] drawing on earlier experience with mouse models,[4] extended the concept of a personalized mutanome vaccine, with an RNA-based poly-neoantigen vaccine, to human therapy. They used exome sequencing to compare melanoma cells with normal cell DNA and identified mutations in the tumour cells. These were studied to predict the mutations that would be expected to result in peptides with high affinity to class II and class I human leucocyte antigen (HLA) molecules, i.e. those that were most likely to be presented effectively to the immune system. They evaluated levels of expression of mutation-encoding RNA. Their selection process was therefore based on neoantigens predicted to generate immunogenic peptides with relatively high levels of transcription. The selected mutations were engineered to make patient-specific synthetic RNA vaccines encoding, usually, 10 neoantigens using clinical grade manufacturing systems. These were injected into lymph nodes and were shown to be translated and to generate immune responses. The clinical rate of new metastatic events in treated patients appeared to be reduced by the mutanome RNA vaccines (Figure 9.3) although some evidence of resistant clonal outgrowth was seen.[8]

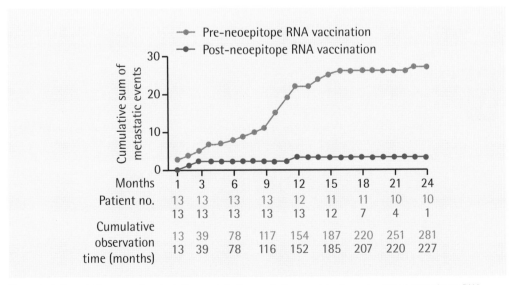

Figure 9.3 Cumulative sum of metastatic events before and after receipt of a personalized neoepitope RNA vaccine. A substantial reduction in metastatic events was seen ($p<0.05$) (adapted from Sahin et al.[8]).

Combined oncolytic virus and neoantigen library approaches

In our laboratories we have sought to generate vaccines of high immunogenicity with broad antigenic coverage by generating cDNA libraries from tumour and normal cell DNA in immunogenic oncolytic viruses.[9,10] This brings together two immunotherapeutic strategies:

- The potential for oncolytic viruses to act as potent non-specific stimulants of immune system response to cancer.

- The potential of cDNA libraries to generate a portfolio of powerfully immunogenic antigens to present to the immune system and therefore reduce the risk of resistant clonal growth.

We showed that a cDNA library derived from normal or malignant tissue could be expressed in a highly immunogenic virus: vesicular stomatitis virus. This viral cDNA library vaccine resulted in the cure of established mouse tumours.[9] Such a broad antigenic repertoire was able to reduce the emergence of resistant subpopulations and may be delivered systematically. We have identified the relevant antigenic determinants[10] and potential mechanisms of neoantigenicity.[11] When cellular cDNA was cloned into vesicular stomatitis virus, viral species emerged with truncated forms of the protein-coding sequences. Truncated cDNA was more effective than full-length cDNA in making effective viral vaccine treatments and had a distinctive immunological effect. These findings may underpin a new clinical vaccine strategy and demonstrate an additional source of tumour neoantigen portfolios for novel vaccine strategies. The anticancer effect of the vaccine is enhanced by ICPIs.[12] The thrust of our future research will be to use the viral library strategy that may be safely used in viruses in the clinic and to combine these as vaccines with non-specific immunotherapies.

Conclusion

 As we further increase our understanding of the patterns and mechanisms of generation of neoantigen portfolios, we may expect novel therapeutic strategies that bring together non-specific promotion of the immune response using ICPIs with the presentation of appropriate portfolios of tumour neoantigens. These have a sound base in our scientific understanding of the immunobiology of cancer and promise further clinical advances.

References

1   Brudno JN, Kochenderfer JN. Chimeric antigen receptor T-cell therapies for lymphoma. *Nat Rev Clin Oncol* 2018; 15: 31–46.

2   De Plaen E, Lurquin C, Van Pel A, *et al*. Immunogenic (tum-) variants of mouse tumor P815: cloning of the gene of tum-antigen P91A and identification of the tum-mutation. *Proc Natl Acad Sci USA* 1988; 85: 2274–8.

3   Matsushita H, Vesely MD, Koboldt DC, *et al*. Cancer exome analysis reveals a T-cell-dependent mechanism of cancer immunoediting. *Nature* 2012; 482: 400–4.

4   Castle JC, Kreiter S, Diekmann J, *et al*. Exploiting the mutanome for tumor vaccination. *Cancer Res* 2012; 72: 1081–91.

5   Saini SK, Rekers N, Hadrup SR. Novel tools to assist neoepitope targeting in personalized cancer immunotherapy. *Ann Oncol* 2017; 28 (suppl 12): xii3–10.

6   Snyder A, Makarov V, Merghoub T, *et al*. Genetic basis for clinical response to CTLA-4 blockade in melanoma. *N Engl J Med* 2014; 371: 2189–99.

7   Alexandrov LB, Nik-Zainal S, Wedge DC, *et al*. Signatures of mutational processes in human cancer. *Nature* 2013; 500: 415–21.

8   Sahin U, Derhovanessian E, Miller M, *et al*. Personalized RNA mutanome vaccines mobilize poly-specific therapeutic immunity against cancer. *Nature* 2017; 547: 222–6.

9   Kottke T, Errington F, Pulido J, *et al*. Broad antigenic coverage induced by vaccination with virus-based cDNA libraries cures established tumors. *Nat Med* 2011; 17: 854–9.

10 Pulido J, Kottke T, Thompson J, *et al*. Using virally expressed melanoma cDNA libraries to identify tumor-associated antigens that cure melanoma. *Nat Biotechnol* 2012; 30: 337–43.

11 Kottke T, Shim KG, Alonso-Camino V, *et al*. Immunogenicity of self tumor associated proteins is enhanced through protein truncation. *Mol Ther Oncolytics* 2016; 3: 16030.

12 Ilett E, Kottke T, Thompson J, *et al*. Prime-boost using separate oncolytic viruses in combination with checkpoint blockade improves anti-tumour therapy. *Gene Ther* 2017; 24: 21–30.

10 Genetically–Modified Cell Therapy for Solid Tumours

Amit Samani, David Marc Davies, Sophie Papa

Introduction

Genetically-modified adoptive T cell therapy (ACT) involves the manufacture *ex vivo* of allogeneic or autologous cells genetically engineered to express either a modified T cell receptor (TCR) or a chimeric antigen receptor (CAR). Stunning responses in chemotherapy-refractory haematological malignancies with cluster of differentiation (CD) 19-targeted CARs have brought ACT into the mainstream of haemato-oncology.[1-5] In 2017, a landmark approval was granted by the US Food and Drug Administration for tisagenlecleucel in acute lymphoblastic leukaemia, followed closely by axicabtagene ciloleucel in relapsed or refractory B cell lymphoma. This chapter introduces the history and current clinical development of ACT, focusing on the challenges unique to solid tumours.

The native TCR is a heterodimer (αβ- or γδ-TCRs). αβ-TCRs recognize antigenic peptides bound to human leucocyte antigens (HLAs). These αβ chains associate with a 'CD3 complex' responsible for transducing the intracellular signal (Figure 10.1). Successful activation of a naive T cell requires further activation through co-stimulatory receptors to avoid anergy.[6]

The development of tumour-infiltrating lymphocyte (TIL) therapy in melanoma has established the feasibility of ACT in the clinic.[7] The observation that the majority of TILs, across donors, were targeting the same antigens, melanoma antigen recognized by T cells 1 (MART-1) and gp100, led to the hypothesis that 'universal' TCR clones could be used to treat different patients so long as they expressed the specific HLA haplotype.[8] Cloning the α and β chains from tumour-reactive TILs into a viral vector for introduction into T cells obviates the need for obtaining TILs from every patient individually and allows modification of the TCR (e.g. to increase affinity).[8]

An alternative strategy, avoiding the need for HLA restriction, is to transduce T cells with CARs. CARs are synthetic receptors composed of an extracellular antigen-binding domain, a transmembrane domain and an intracellular signalling domain, designed to deliver T cell activation on antigen engagement (Figure 10.2). The antigen-binding domain most commonly takes the form of a single-chain variable fragment (scFv) derived from an antibody specific to the tumour-associated antigen of choice, but may include other moieties such as natural or chimeric ligands.[9-11]

CAR/TCR ACT has numerous attractive qualities:

- Specificity, so that selection of the right antigen should spare non-expressing tissues.

- The ability to proliferate and persist, such that a single infused dose could have a marked, durable effect.

- Potent cytotoxicity capability.

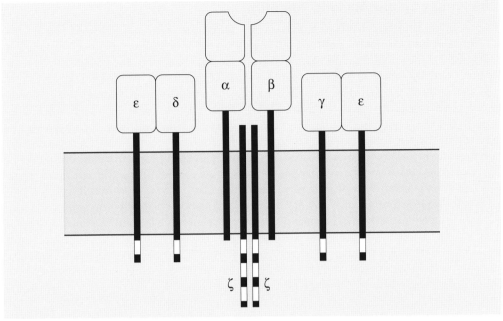

Figure 10.1 Schematic diagram of the structure of the TCR complex. The four monomers and two dimers form an eight-chain complex that incorporates antigen recognition through the α and β chains with transduction of signal 1 to the T cell through the γ, δ, ε and ζ chains.

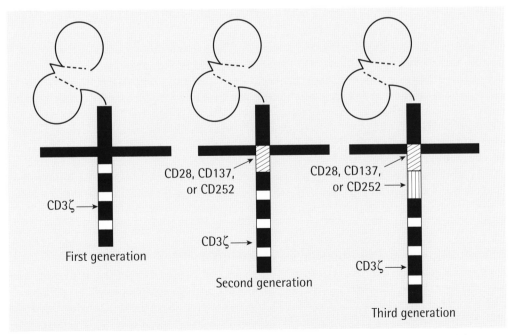

Figure 10.2 Diagram of CAR design incorporating an extracellular antigen-binding domain in series with intracellular signalling components. Evolution from first to third generation has involved the incorporation of co-stimulatory signalling domains to potentiate CAR signalling and T cell activation on antigen engagement.

Challenges unique to solid tumours

Progress in solid tumours has been hampered by some unique challenges. These are best appreciated by imagining the journey of the infused product following administration. First, the cells must traffic to the tumour. Unlike haematological tumours, where the cancerous cells may reside in more 'natural' homing sites (e.g. lymphoid organs), solid tumours may disseminate unpredictably and unusually. Furthermore, they fail to express chemokines matched to the T cell profile and conversely may actually inhibit T cell trafficking. If the product eventually reaches the tumour, it needs to extravasate into the tumour microenvironment. If the cells make it through, the abnormal tumour vasculature poses a physical barrier further compounded by tumour-associated stroma. Once in the tumour microenvironment, many immunosuppressive factors including cells (e.g. regulatory T cells, myeloid-derived suppressor cells), soluble factors (e.g. adenosine, transforming growth factor [TGF]-β), immune checkpoints (e.g. programmed death-ligand 1 [PD-L1], lymphocyte-activation gene [LAG]-3 protein) and a hostile metabolic environment devoid of nutrients, high in lactate and low in oxygen all act to suppress effector T cell mechanisms and induce a state of anergy. Even if all these barriers are overcome, there remains the issue of selecting the optimal antigen to target. Solid tumours unfortunately display marked intra- and inter-tumoural heterogeneity and often share antigens with vital normal structures, thereby increasing the risk of tumour escape or 'on-target, off-organ' toxicity.

Recent developments

TCRs

The first successful trial used engineered MART-1 TCRs and produced responses in two out of 17 patients.[12] This modest success provided proof of concept. In an attempt to boost efficacy a higher-affinity engineered MART-1 TCR was used.[13] The response rate was higher (six out of 20 patients), but novel autoimmune toxicity emerged including rash, vitiligo, and sight and hearing problems, all of which (except vitiligo) resolved with steroids. These results demonstrated that while engineering 'supraphysiological' affinity could improve response, it could also generate novel toxicity through broadening specificity to antigenic peptide epitopes with some sequence homology with the cognate peptide. Nonetheless, the promising efficacy paved the way for other trials targeting antigens including gp100, carcinoembryonic antigen (CEA), NY-ESO-1 and melanoma-associated antigen 3 (MAGE-A3), all of which have produced responses but with some toxicity due to cross-reactivity with similar epitopes.[14–16] Of note, a trial using a TCR against NY-ESO-1 in patients with heavily pretreated refractory synovial cell sarcoma and melanoma produced responses in nine out of 17 patients, with no dose-limiting toxicity.[16] NY-ESO-1 is found in various high-prevalence epithelial cancers; there are currently 22 active or recruiting trials using TCRs against this antigen.

CARs

By targeting cell surface antigens, independently of the major histocompatibility complex (MHC), CAR therapy provides an alternative strategy. Initial trials with CAR T cells used first generation constructs without co-stimulatory domains (Figure 10.2). Efficacy was limited and investigations revealed poor proliferation and persistence of CARs *in vivo*.[17–19] Incorporation of co-stimulatory domains into the intracellular region of a CAR construct in preclinical models provided evidence of superior proliferation and persistence.[20,21] In 2008, Pule *et al.*[22] transduced Epstein–Barr virus-specific T cells with a GD2-specific first generation CAR. The viral specificity of the transduced T cell population ensured the delivery of co-stimulation to the CAR T cell alongside the CD3 signal

1 delivered through the CAR itself. This approach resulted in the first clinical evidence of efficacy and persistence of CAR T cells. Building a second generation CAR with CD28 co-stimulation as part of the apparatus improved persistence and expansion of CAR T cells in the clinic in 2011, cementing the engineering approach in ongoing CAR design (Figure 10.2).[23] Clinical translation was hampered in 2011, when a fatal serious adverse event occurred in a first-in-human CAR T cell trial. A patient with colorectal cancer was treated intravenously with 10×10^{10} third generation CAR T cells directed against human epidermal growth factor receptor 2 (HER2).[24] Acute respiratory distress rapidly developed. Autopsy confirmed low-level HER2 expression in the pulmonary epithelium. This was a stark warning of the potential for on-target, off-tumour toxicity and understandably led to caution in applying CAR therapy to solid tumours.

Incorporation of lymphodepleting doses of chemotherapy to transiently clear the lymphocyte pool in the patient prior to T cell infusion was a key step in improving the efficacy of TIL therapy for melanoma.[7,25] This approach has been successfully extrapolated to haematological CAR T cell studies, albeit at the risk of escalated high adverse event rates due to amplified cytokine release syndrome and neurological toxicity. Nonetheless, results in haematological cancers have fuelled interest in solid tumours, resulting in use in clinical development of much lower doses (e.g. between 10^4 and 10^8 cells) and cautious dose escalations in first-in-human trials. Encouraging efficacy has recently been seen against targets including prostate-specific membrane antigen (producing a partial response in two out of five patients with prostate cancer),[26] CD133 plus epidermal growth factor (EGF) receptor (producing a partial response lasting 13 months in a patient with cholangiocarcinoma),[27] interleukin-13 receptor subunit α2 (IL-13Rα2) (producing a complete response in a patient with multifocal refractory glioblastoma)[28] and a HER2-directed CAR (producing one partial response and prolonged stable disease in several patients with sarcomas).[29] There are many active trials still recruiting or yet to report, and even more yet to start.

Future directions

The field of adoptive cellular therapy for solid tumours is still in its infancy. There is a huge volume of preclinical and translational research focused on optimizing CAR/TCR design, improving manufacturing techniques and overcoming logistical hurdles for broad application in the clinic. CARs are being engineered to express specific chemokine receptors,[30] secrete enzymes to digest the extracellular matrix,[31] and express engineered receptors that bind to otherwise inhibitory ligands (e.g. PD-L1) and transduce a stimulatory signal.[32] Furthermore, CAR T cells that express multiple antigen-targeting moieties are being developed either to overcome intra- and inter-tumoural heterogeneity or to enhance safety (e.g. by using a Boolean logic gated system where both targets must engage in order for the CAR to function, thereby reducing the chance of cytotoxicity against normal tissue only expressing one antigen).[33] Safety controls such as 'suicide switches'[34] or the use of RNA transduction (producing only transient CAR expression)[35] are being incorporated to reduce concern over uncontrollable toxicity.

For engineered TCRs, we may see a shift towards patient-specific neoantigen-based constructs. In many tumours, TIL effectiveness stems from neoantigen-specific clones.[8] As sequencing and neoantigen prediction become quicker and cheaper it may be feasible to engineer TCRs for truly personalized therapy.

Route of delivery may have an impact.[28,36] Alternatively, combination therapy is likely to produce a synergistic effect. In a recent CAR trial targeting EGF receptor variant III in glioblastoma, evaluation of the tumour microenvironment revealed increased expression of inhibitory molecules and infiltration by regulatory T cells, suggesting that CAR T cells can traffic to the tumour and mediate cytotoxicity but that adaptive resistance mechanisms enable tumours to avoid elimination.[37] Blocking programmed cell death protein 1 (PD-1)-mediated CAR T cell inhibition in a mesothelioma model counters intrinsic resistance.[38] In a patient with diffuse large B cell lymphoma, pembrolizumab treatment after early progression post-CD19 CAR T cell treatment promoted alternative CAR T cell clones, potentially explaining subsequent disease response.[39] These results certainly suggest hypotheses regarding combination therapy in the future.

Conclusion

Genetically-modified T cell therapy is an established therapy for CD19 haematological cancers. Solid tumour advances are now gathering pace. This form of 'living drug' is fraught with challenges, from procurement and manufacturing through to toxicity. The different permutations and combinations are innumerable; however, as with many great breakthroughs in medicine, serendipity is likely to play a part. Given the current level of effort and enthusiasm, it is only a matter of time before we stumble upon the optimum combination of factors to mediate a paradigm shift in treatment.

References

1 Brentjens RJ, Davila ML, Rivière I, et al. CD19-targeted T cells rapidly induce molecular remissions in adults with chemotherapy-refractory acute lymphoblastic leukemia. *Sci Transl Med* 2013; 5: 177ra38.

2 Davila ML, Rivière I, Wang X, et al. Efficacy and toxicity management of 19–28z CAR T cell therapy in B cell acute lymphoblastic leukemia. *Sci Transl Med* 2014; 6: 224ra25.

3 Kochenderfer JN, Dudley ME, Kassim SH, et al. Chemotherapy-refractory diffuse large B-cell lymphoma and indolent B-cell malignancies can be effectively treated with autologous T cells expressing an anti-CD19 chimeric antigen receptor. *J Clin Oncol* 2015; 33: 540–9.

4 Lee DW, Kochenderfer JN, Stetler-Stevenson M, et al. T cells expressing CD19 chimeric antigen receptors for acute lymphoblastic leukaemia in children and young adults: a phase 1 dose-escalation trial. *Lancet* 2015; 385: 517–28.

5 Maude SL, Frey N, Shaw PA, et al. Chimeric antigen receptor T cells for sustained remissions in leukemia. *N Engl J Med* 2014; 371: 1507–17.

6 Chen L, Flies DB. Molecular mechanisms of T cell co-stimulation and co-inhibition. *Nat Rev Immunol* 2013; 13: 227–42.

7 Dudley ME, Wunderlich JR, Robbins PF, et al. Cancer regression and autoimmunity in patients after clonal repopulation with antitumor lymphocytes. *Science* 2002; 298: 850–4.

8 Johnson LA, June CH. Driving gene-engineered T cell immunotherapy of cancer. *Cell Res* 2017; 27: 38–58.

9 Davies DM, Foster J, Van Der Stegen SJ, et al. Flexible targeting of ErbB dimers that drive tumorigenesis by using genetically engineered T cells. *Mol Med* 2012; 18: 565–76.

10 Eshhar Z, Waks T, Gross G, Schindler DG. Specific activation and targeting of cytotoxic lymphocytes through chimeric single chains consisting of antibody-binding domains and the gamma or zeta subunits of the immunoglobulin and T-cell receptors. *Proc Natl Acad Sci USA* 1993; 90: 720–4.

11 Srivastava S, Riddell SR. Engineering CAR-T cells: design concepts. *Trends Immunol* 2015; 36: 494–502.

12 Hughes MS, Yu YY, Dudley ME, *et al.* Transfer of a TCR gene derived from a patient with a marked antitumor response conveys highly active T-cell effector functions. *Hum Gene Ther* 2005; 16: 457–72.

13 Johnson LA, Morgan RA, Dudley ME, *et al.* Gene therapy with human and mouse T-cell receptors mediates cancer regression and targets normal tissues expressing cognate antigen. *Blood* 2009; 114: 535–46.

14 Morgan RA, Chinnasamy N, Abate-Daga D, *et al.* Cancer regression and neurological toxicity following anti-MAGE-A3 TCR gene therapy. *J Immunother* 2013; 36: 133–51.

15 Parkhurst MR, Yang JC, Langan RC, *et al.* T cells targeting carcinoembryonic antigen can mediate regression of metastatic colorectal cancer but induce severe transient colitis. *Mol Ther* 2011; 19: 620–6.

16 Robbins PF, Morgan RA, Feldman SA, *et al.* Tumor regression in patients with metastatic synovial cell sarcoma and melanoma using genetically engineered lymphocytes reactive with NY-ESO-1. *J Clin Oncol* 2011; 29: 917–24.

17 Kershaw MH, Westwood JA, Parker LL, *et al.* A phase I study on adoptive immunotherapy using gene-modified T cells for ovarian cancer. *Clin Cancer Res* 2006; 12: 6106–15.

18 Lamers CH, Sleijfer S, Vulto AG, *et al.* Treatment of metastatic renal cell carcinoma with autologous T-lymphocytes genetically retargeted against carbonic anhydrase IX: first clinical experience. *J Clin Oncol* 2006; 24: e20–2.

19 Park JR, Digiusto DL, Slovak M, *et al.* Adoptive transfer of chimeric antigen receptor re-directed cytolytic T lymphocyte clones in patients with neuroblastoma. *Mol Ther* 2007; 15: 825–33.

20 Carpenito C, Milone MC, Hassan R, *et al.* Control of large, established tumor xenografts with genetically retargeted human T cells containing CD28 and CD137 domains. *Proc Natl Acad Sci USA* 2009; 106: 3360–5.

21 Maher J, Brentjens RJ, Gunset G, *et al.* Human T-lymphocyte cytotoxicity and proliferation directed by a single chimeric TCRzeta/CD28 receptor. *Nat Biotechnol* 2002; 20: 70–5.

22 Pule MA, Savoldo B, Myers GD, *et al.* Virus-specific T cells engineered to coexpress tumor-specific receptors: persistence and antitumor activity in individuals with neuroblastoma. *Nat Med* 2008; 14: 1264–70.

23 Savoldo B, Ramos CA, Liu E, *et al.* CD28 costimulation improves expansion and persistence of chimeric antigen receptor-modified T cells in lymphoma patients. *J Clin Invest* 2011; 121: 1822–6.

24 Morgan RA, Yang JC, Kitano M, *et al.* Case report of a serious adverse event following the administration of T cells transduced with a chimeric antigen receptor recognizing *ERBB2*. *Mol Ther* 2010; 18: 843–51.

25 Dudley ME, Wunderlich JR, Yang JC, *et al.* Adoptive cell transfer therapy following non-myeloablative but lymphodepleting chemotherapy for the treatment of patients with refractory metastatic melanoma. *J Clin Oncol* 2005; 23: 2346–57.

26 Junghans RP, Ma Q, Rathore R, *et al.* Phase I trial of anti-PSMA designer CAR-T cells in prostate cancer: possible role for interacting interleukin 2-T cell pharmacodynamics as a determinant of clinical response. *Prostate* 2016; 76: 1257–70.

27 Feng KC, Guo YL, Liu Y, *et al.* Cocktail treatment with EGFR-specific and CD133-specific chimeric antigen receptor-modified T cells in a patient with advanced cholangiocarcinoma. *J Hematol Oncol* 2017; 10: 4.

28 Brown CE, Alizadeh D, Starr R, *et al*. Regression of glioblastoma after chimeric antigen receptor T-cell therapy. *N Engl J Med* 2016; 375: 2561–9.

29 Ahmed N, Brawley V, Hegde M, *et al*. HER2-specific chimeric antigen receptor-modified virus-specific T cells for progressive glioblastoma: a phase 1 dose-escalation trial. *JAMA Oncol* 2017; 3: 1094–101.

30 Craddock JA, Lu A, Bear A, *et al*. Enhanced tumor trafficking of GD2 chimeric antigen receptor T cells by expression of the chemokine receptor CCR2b. *J Immunother* 2010; 33: 780–8.

31 Caruana I, Savoldo B, Hoyos V, *et al*. Heparanase promotes tumor infiltration and antitumor activity of CAR-redirected T lymphocytes. *Nat Med* 2015; 21: 524–9.

32 Liu X, Ranganathan R, Jiang S, *et al*. A chimeric switch-receptor targeting PD1 augments the efficacy of second-generation CAR T cells in advanced solid tumors. *Cancer Res* 2016; 76: 1578–90.

33 Davies DM, Maher J. Gated chimeric antigen receptor T-cells: the next logical step in reducing toxicity? *Transl Cancer Res* 2016; 5 (suppl 1): S61–5.

34 Straathof KC, Pule MA, Yotnda P, *et al*. An inducible caspase 9 safety switch for T-cell therapy. *Blood* 2005; 105: 4247–54.

35 Rabinovich PM, Komarovskaya ME, Wrzesinski SH, *et al*. Chimeric receptor mRNA transfection as a tool to generate antineoplastic lymphocytes. *Hum Gene Ther* 2009; 20: 51–61.

36 Papa S, van Schalkwyk M, Maher J. Clinical evaluation of ErbB-targeted CAR T-cells, following intracavity delivery in patients with ErbB-expressing solid tumors. *Methods Mol Biol* 2015; 1317: 365–82.

37 O'Rourke DM, Nasrallah MP, Desai A, *et al*. A single dose of peripherally infused EGFRvIII-directed CAR T cells mediates antigen loss and induces adaptive resistance in patients with recurrent glioblastoma. *Sci Transl Med* 2017; 9: pii eaaa0984.

38 Cherkassky L, Morello A, Villena-Vargas J, *et al*. Human CAR T cells with cell-intrinsic PD-1 checkpoint blockade resist tumor-mediated inhibition. *J Clin Invest* 2016; 126: 3130–44.

39 Chong EA, Melenhorst JJ, Lacey SF, *et al*. PD-1 blockade modulates chimeric antigen receptor (CAR)-modified T cells: refueling the CAR. *Blood* 2017; 129: 1039–41.

Further reading

• Eyquem J, Mansilla-Soto J, Giavridis T, *et al*. Targeting a CAR to the *TRAC* locus with CRISPR/Cas9 enhances tumour rejection. *Nature* 2017; 543: 113–17.

• Kagoya Y, Tanaka S, Guo T, *et al*. A novel chimeric antigen receptor containing a JAK-STAT signaling domain mediates superior antitumor effects. *Nat Med* 2018; 24: 352–9.

• Louis CU, Salvodo B, Dotti G, *et al*. Antitumour activity and long-term fate of chimeric antigen receptor-positive T cells in patients with neuroblastoma. *Blood* 2011; 118: 6050–6.

• Rosenberg S, Restifo N. Adoptive cell transfer as personalized immunotherapy for human cancer. *Science* 2015; 348: 62–8.

• Sadelain M, Rivière I, Riddell S. Therapeutic T cell engineering. *Nature* 2017; 545: 423–31.

11 Adoptive T Cell Therapy for Haematological Malignancies

Reuben Benjamin, Charlotte Graham

Introduction

The anticancer potential of the immune system has long been recognized in haematological malignancies, with allogeneic stem cell transplantation and donor lymphocyte infusions now established as standards of care for acute myeloid leukaemia (AML), acute lymphoblastic leukaemia (ALL) and some types of lymphomas. In addition, immunomodulatory drugs and monoclonal antibodies that trigger antibody-dependent cell-mediated cytotoxicity have been shown to be effective treatments for multiple myeloma and B cell lymphomas (e.g. B cell non-Hodgkin lymphoma [B-NHL]). The accessibility of bone marrow and lymph nodes (the predominant sites of haematological tumours) to circulating immune cells, as well as their susceptibility to immune cell-mediated killing, makes them an obvious target for adoptive T cell therapy (ACT). It was, however, the discovery that T lymphocytes could be retargeted to tumour cells, independently of the major histocompatibility complex (MHC), using chimeric antigen receptors (CARs) that fuelled interest in the field of ACT for haematological malignancies.

A CAR T cell is an artificial T cell receptor (TCR) consisting of an antigen-binding domain derived from a monoclonal antibody (single-chain variable fragment), an activation domain (cluster of differentiation [CD] 3ζ) and a co-stimulatory domain (typically CD28 or CD4–1bb).[1] The target antigen is generally expressed strongly and homogenously on the surface of tumour cells, with little or no expression on normal cells, and ideally plays a role in tumour survival.

Results from CAR T cell trials in haematological malignancies

CD19, an antigen expressed on normal B lymphocytes and B cell lineage malignancies, was the target of the initial CAR T cell products, given its relative specificity and strong expression in chronic lymphocytic leukaemia (CLL), B cell ALL (B-ALL) and B-NHL.

Initial studies with first generation CAR T cells lacking a co-stimulatory domain failed to show persistence of the CAR T cell *in vivo*, or any clinical activity. The first reports of the successful use of CD19 CAR T cells came in 2011 from groups led by Michel Sadelain, Carl June and Steven Rosenberg using second generation CAR T cells in CLL, B-ALL and follicular NHL.[2-4] These studies highlighted the importance of having a co-stimulatory domain within the CAR T cell construct and the need to use lymphodepleting drugs to facilitate CAR T cell expansion. After these early promising results a number of other phase I studies were conducted in relapsed paediatric and adult B-ALL patients showing highly impressive complete response rates of 70–90% irrespective of which CD19 CAR T cell was used. The long-term outcome from CD19 CAR T cell treatment was confirmed by the Determine Efficacy and Safety of Tisagenlecleucel in Pediatric Patients with Relapsed and Refractory B-Cell ALL (ELIANA) study, which showed an overall remission rate of 81%, event-free survival of 50% and overall survival of 76%, 12 months after CAR T cell treatment in patients <21 years with relapsed B-ALL.[5] Although the initial strategy was to offer an allogeneic stem cell transplant as consolidation following CAR T cell therapy, it became clear that CAR T cells could persist for many months (especially CD4-1bb-based CARs), with B cell aplasia as a surrogate marker of ongoing clinical activity, thus avoiding the need for subsequent allogeneic stem cell transplant and making CD19 CAR T cell therapy a potential stand-alone curative treatment for relapsed B-ALL.

The results of CD19 CAR T cell treatment in high grade B-NHL have been very encouraging, with an overall response rate of 82% in relapsed/refractory diffuse large B cell lymphoma (DLBCL).[6] The Phase I–II Multicenter Study Evaluating Axicabtagene Ciloleucel in Subjects with Refractory Aggressive Non-Hodgkin Lymphoma (ZUMA-1) achieved a complete response rate of 54%, with 40% of patients remaining in complete response at a median follow-up of 15 months.[6] Similar efficacy was seen with a different CD19 CAR T cell product in the Study of Efficacy and Safety of Tisagenlecleucel in Adult DLBCL Patients (JULIET), which had an overall response rate of 53%, with 40% of patients achieving a complete response.[7] After these impressive clinical trial results the two CD19 CAR T cell products tisagenlecleucel and axicabtagene ciloleucel received US Food and Drug Administration approval in 2017 for relapsed/refractory paediatric/young adult B-ALL and DLBCL, respectively. Tisagenlecleucel was subsequently also approved for DLBCL; approval by the European Medicines Agency is expected in 2018.

The first real evidence that CAR T cell therapy could be effective for targets other than CD19 came from trials in multiple myeloma using a B cell membrane antigen (BCMA)-targeted CAR T cell. Two phase I trials using different BCMA CAR T cell products and targeting heavily pretreated patients showed spectacular response rates of 94–100%, with a high proportion of deep responses (complete response and stringent complete response).[8,9] The follow-up to date, however, remains short. A number of other CAR T cell trials in haematological malignancies are underway targeting CD22 in B-ALL, CD123 in AML, signalling lymphocytic activation molecule F7 (CS1) in myeloma and CD3 in T cell NHL. Despite the impressive response rates to CAR T cell therapy, the long-term outcomes remain unclear outside the paediatric/young adult B-ALL setting. It is hoped the picture will become clearer within a few years when longer follow-up data are available.

Toxicity of CAR T cell therapy

What has also emerged from the early CAR T cell trials has been a side effect profile common to many CAR T cell products. The major side effects observed to date include cytokine release syndrome (CRS) and neurotoxicity.[10] CRS occurs in the majority of patients treated with CAR T cells and arises as a result of activation of CAR T cells after encounter with their target antigen. A range of cytokines and chemokines including interleukin (IL)-2, interferon (IFN)-γ, tumour necrosis factor (TNF)-α, granulocyte macrophage colony-stimulating factor (GM-CSF) and IL-6 are released by activated CAR T cells as well as bystander immune cells such as monocytes and macrophages leading to constitutional symptoms of fevers, malaise and myalgia, as well as cardiac, respiratory, renal, liver and neurological dysfunction. The severity of CRS is dependent on the disease burden, presence of comorbidities, type of CAR T cell product and infused cell dose. Management of CRS comprises the use of antipyretics, anti-IL-6 pathway inhibitors such as tocilizumab, steroids, antibiotics to treat coexisting infections and organ support on the ITU if appropriate.

Neurotoxicity is a potentially debilitating side effect of CAR T cell therapy and has been observed in at least a third of treated patients. Symptoms may include confusion, aphasia, somnolence, agitation, tremors and seizures. The pathophysiology remains poorly understood although it is thought to be cytokine mediated. The majority of cases recover spontaneously but rare cases of fatal cerebral oedema have been reported. Treatment of neurotoxicity is generally supportive; steroids are used for more severe symptoms and antiepileptics are used in the event of seizures. Tocilizumab is recommended if there is concurrent CRS. Close monitoring on the ITU is essential, with management guided by a neurologist and appropriate investigations performed (e.g. EEG, MRI brain, lumbar puncture).

Other side effects seen following CAR T cell therapy include macrophage activation syndrome and B cell aplasia. Macrophage activation syndrome presents with high serum ferritin levels, grade 3 or higher organ toxicity, cytopenias, haemophagocytosis in bone marrow and high cytokine levels. While the picture may overlap with CRS it is typically resistant to anti-IL-6 and steroid treatment. A long-term consequence of CD19 and BCMA CAR T cell therapy is the development of prolonged B cell aplasia and consequent risk of infections requiring treatment with antibiotics and prophylactic use of intravenous immunoglobulins.

Tumour escape following CAR T cell treatment

Despite the impressive early efficacy of CD19 CAR T cell therapy in B cell malignancies, tumour escape does occur through a variety of mechanisms.[11] These include CAR T cell exhaustion and/ or lack of persistence, target antigen downregulation, the requirement for CAR T cells to home to tumour sanctuary sites particularly outside the bone marrow, and the inhibitory effect of the tumour microenvironment. Strategies to overcome these resistance mechanisms are currently being evaluated including the use of CARs engineered to improve persistence, use of dual antigen-targeted CARs and concurrent use of immune checkpoint inhibitors.

ACT beyond CAR T cells

While CAR T cells have undoubtedly been the star performers in the field of ACT, a number of other immune effector cells are also being evaluated in clinical trials including New York oesophageal squamous cell carcinoma-1 (NY-ESO-1) -targeted TCRs for myeloma (ClinicalTrials.gov NCT03168438), allogeneic natural killer cells for AML after haploidentical stem cell transplant (ClinicalTrials.gov NCT01904136), γδ T cells for AML (ClinicalTrials.gov NCT03533816) and T regulatory cells for chronic graft vs host disease (ClinicalTrials.gov NCT02749084). With advances in cell manufacturing processes, improved trial design and additional gene modification of immune effector cells to enhance potency, further progress is likely to be seen in the field of ACT for haematological malignancies.

Challenges in delivering CAR T cell treatment

The spectacular success of CAR T cell therapy in B cell malignancies and the approval of tisagenlecleucel and axicabtagene ciloleucel for B-ALL and DLBCL have focused attention on the ability of healthcare systems globally to deliver this potentially toxic and expensive therapy.[12] Unique challenges have arisen as a consequence of the publicity surrounding this field, accompanied by unrealistic expectations on the part of patients, treating physicians, academics, the pharmaceutical industry and governments. The need to involve the ITU and multiple other specialties poses a burden on most healthcare systems even in the developed world. A new generation of 'cell therapists' will have to be trained comprising clinicians, nurses, pharmacists, cell therapy laboratory staff and quality managers. The challenge for the field is enormous, but the potential impact for patients with terminal cancer is even greater.

References

1 Sadelain M, Brentjens R, Rivière I. The basic principles of chimeric antigen receptor design. *Cancer Discov* 2018; 3: 388–98.

2 Brentjens RJ, Rivière I, Park JH, *et al.* Safety and persistence of adoptively transferred autologous CD19-targeted T cells in patients with relapsed or chemotherapy refractory B-cell leukemias. *Blood* 2011; 118: 4817–28.

3 Porter DL, Levine BL, Kalos M, *et al.* Chimeric antigen receptor-modified T cells in chronic lymphoid leukemia. *N Engl J Med* 2011; 365: 725–33.

4 Kochenderfer JN, Wilson WH, Janik JE, *et al.* Eradication of B-lineage cells and regression of lymphoma in a patient treated with autologous T cells genetically engineered to recognize CD19. *Blood* 2010; 116: 4099–102.

5 Maude SL, Laetsch TW, Buechner J, *et al.* Tisagenlecleucel in children and young adults with B-cell lymphoblastic leukemia. *N Engl J Med* 2018; 378: 439–48.

6 Neelapu SS, Locke FL, Bartlett NL, *et al.* Axicabtagene ciloleucel CAR T-cell therapy in refractory large B-cell lymphoma. *N Engl J Med* 2017; 377: 2531–44.

7 Schuster SJ, Svoboda J, Chong EA, *et al.* Chimeric antigen receptor T cells in refractory B-cell lymphomas. *N Engl J Med* 2017; 377: 2545–54.

8 Berdeja JG, Lin Y, Raje NS, *et al.* First-in-human multicenter study of bb2121 anti-BCMA CAR T-cell therapy for relapsed/refractory multiple myeloma: updated results. *J Clin Oncol* 2017; 35 (15 suppl): 3010.

9 Fan F, Zhao W, Liu J, *et al.* Durable remissions with BCMA specific chimeric antigen receptor (CAR)-modified T cells in patients with refractory/relapsed multiple myeloma. Presented at: American Society of Clinical Oncology annual meeting, June 2017. Abstract LBA3001.

10 Neelapu SS, Tummala S, Kebriaei P, *et al.* Chimeric antigen receptor T-cell therapy: assessment and management of toxicities. *Nat Rev Clin Oncol* 2018; 15: 47–62.

11 Gardner R, Wu D, Cherian S, *et al.* Acquisition of a CD19-negative myeloid phenotype allows immune escape of *MLL*-rearranged B-ALL from CD19 CAR-T-cell therapy. *Blood* 2016; 127: 2406–10.

12 Buechner J, Kersten MJ, Fuchs M, *et al.* Chimeric antigen receptor T-cell therapy: practical considerations for implementation in Europe. *HemaSphere* 2018; 2: e18.

12 Tumour-Infiltrating Lymphocytes

Magnus Pedersen, Robert Hawkins, Fiona Thistlethwaite

Introduction

Adoptive T cell therapy (ACT) is treatment with immune cells collected from a patient, then grown and manipulated in a laboratory and subsequently administered back to the patient. The aim is to induce a specific anti-tumour response, making ACT a highly personalized form of immunotherapy. ACT takes two main forms:

- T cells that have natural anti-tumour reactivity, for example tumour-infiltrating lymphocyte (TIL) therapy.
- T cells that are gene-modified to direct an anti-tumour response, for example chimeric antigen receptor therapy.

This chapter focuses on the use of lymphocytes that have natural anti-tumour reactivity, specifically TIL therapy.

Background

TILs are naturally occurring cells that have the ability to infiltrate tissue with the purpose of specifically recognizing malignant cells and eliminating them. They do so either by recognizing antigens shared by the patient and the malignant cells (self antigens)[1] or by recognizing tumour-specific antigens (neoantigens), the latter being present due to somatic mutations of the malignant cells.[2] TILs are generated as part of an adaptive immune response to the cancer when considered foreign by the immune system. In some cases, emerging tumours can develop means of avoiding elimination by the immune system, and clinically detectable cancer disease will develop.[3] ACT with TILs exploits the fact that the adaptive immune system has already generated specific TILs against the cancer that can potentially recognize and eliminate the cancer cells but are being prevented from doing so. There may be several reasons why TILs are not able to eliminate malignant cells; some of these can be diminished or bypassed through conditioning and stimulating treatment in relation to ACT with TILs. This, and the historical development of ACT with TILs, will be elaborated upon in this chapter.

Recent developments

Development of TIL therapy

In the 1980s, Rosenberg *et al.*[4] discovered in a murine model that TILs in combination with the T cell growth factor interleukin (IL)-2 were superior to lymphokine-activated killer cells in killing cancer cells and seemed to retain specificity for the tumour from which they were derived. In the first TIL pilot study, 12 patients with metastatic melanoma or renal cell carcinoma (RCC) were treated with IL-2-expanded TILs and subsequent IL-2 stimulation with or without lymphodepleting cyclophosphamide chemotherapy prior to TIL infusion. Two patients in the cyclophosphamide group achieved a partial response.[5] Since then, increased knowledge about TILs has led to remarkable progress in developing methods to expand them *ex vivo*, improving lymphodepleting conditioning and optimizing stimulation with IL-2. In 2011, Rosenberg *et al.*[6] published the final analysis of three sequential clinical trials, demonstrating a response rate of 49–72%; 22% of metastatic melanoma patients achieved a complete response. When treated with TILs preceded by lymphodepleting chemotherapy and followed by high-dose bolus infusions of IL-2 the majority of the complete responses persisted years after treatment. The most commonly used TIL therapy regimen today arises from this work and comparable studies, and has primarily been investigated in the setting of malignant melanoma. An overview of this regimen and the rationale behind treating patients with ACT with TILs is given below.

Current practice in TIL therapy

In terms of TIL expansion, the general approach is to use excised autologous tumour tissue for *ex vivo* growth and activation of TILs in a laboratory before infusion. The tumour tissue is divided into fragments that are initially cultured with IL-2. Further growth to reach treatment numbers (billions of cells) is done through stimulation with irradiated allogeneic feeder cells (peripheral blood mononuclear cells that cannot divide and secrete cytokines that stimulate TIL growth), an anti-cluster of differentiation (CD) 3 antibody (for stimulation of the TILs and the feeder cells) and high concentrations of IL-2. During expansion, TILs may be selected on the basis of their ability to recognize autologous tumour *in vitro* (selected TILs) or be expanded, with emphasis on the TILs spending a minimum of time in culture (young/selected TILs).[7,8] The general consensus is that the CD8+ effector memory cells are the most important T cell subset in terms of achieving tumour regression in malignant melanoma (although conflicting findings have been reported[9]), while in non-melanoma it is less clear.

Lymphodepletion is the destruction of lymphocytes including T cells. Lymphodepleting conditioning chemotherapy prior to TIL therapy has been shown to increase the objective response rate.[10] Several mechanisms of action have been proposed through the study of murine models: (1) infused TILs are more likely to expand and engraft; (2) there is decreased competition with endogenous T cells for antigen interaction; (3) immunosuppressive regulatory T cells are depleted; and (4) cells that are competing for host homeostatic cytokines are removed.[8]

IL-2 is a cytokine with several functions in the immune response.[11] It has been used in the treatment of malignant melanoma since the 1980s, achieving a response rate of 15% and a complete response rate of 4–5%.[12] The rationale of administering IL-2 after TIL infusion is to activate and promote continued growth of the TILs.[8]

In overview, the most commonly used regimen of ACT with TILs consists of initial lymphodepleting chemotherapy administered for 7 days prior to TIL infusion comprising an initial 2 days of cyclophosphamide treatment (60 mg/kg per day) followed by 5 days of fludarabine treatment (25 mg/m² per day, maximum dosage of 50 mg) (Figure 12.1). Lymphodepletion is followed by infusion of billions of TILs. High numbers of infused TILs have been shown to be associated with a clinical response in patients with malignant melanoma.[13] TIL infusion is followed by IL-2 stimulation. The most widely used regimen consists of high-dose bolus IL-2 (720,000 IU/kg) every 8 h for a total of 15 doses or fewer depending on toxicities. While there seems to be a consensus regarding the lymphodepleting conditioning preceding TIL infusion, the exact design of the subsequent IL-2 stimulation regimen is more unclear,[14] and altered IL-2 stimulation regimens have been tested. A reduced IL-2 dosage has been shown to reduce toxicity, both in a low-dose subcutaneous regimen[15] and with an intermediate dose using a decrescendo regimen,[16] achieving a partial response in two out of six treated patients and responses similar to those seen with the high-dose bolus IL-2 regimen, respectively.

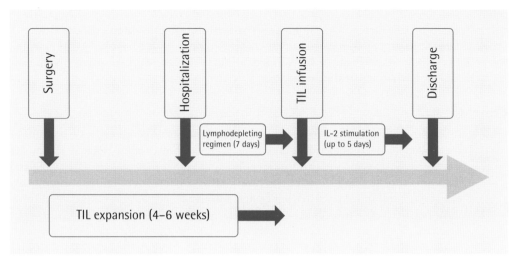

Figure 12.1 Overview of TIL scheme.

TIL therapy in solid tumours

ACT with TILs has previously been investigated in cancers other than malignant melanoma, including ovarian cancer, RCC, non-small-cell lung carcinoma (NSCLC) and glioma.[7] These older trials were typically performed without lymphodepleting conditioning, with suboptimal regimens of IL-2 stimulation and earlier methods of TIL expansion leading to lower numbers of infused TILs.

In recent years, clinical trials investigating ACT with TILs in malignancies other than melanoma have been scarce. Most spectacular was a study performed by Stevanović et al.[17] in patients with metastatic cervical cancer with human papilloma virus (HPV)-targeted TILs which achieved three responses in nine patients, two of whom had a complete response. Several single-diagnosis clinical trials have been initiated in ovarian cancer (ClinicalTrials.gov NCT02482090 and NCT03287674), RCC (ClinicalTrials.gov NCT02926053), head and neck cancer (ClinicalTrials.gov NCT03083873), cervical cancer (ClinicalTrials.gov NCT03108495), NSCLC (ClinicalTrials.gov NCT03215810 and NCT03419559) and mesothelioma (ClinicalTrials.gov NCT02414945). There are also a few clinical trials investigating ACT with TILs in multiple malignancies (ClinicalTrials.gov NCT01462903, NCT01174121 and NCT03296137). These trials span from ACT with TILs in a classical setting to altered regimens of IL-2 stimulation and combination regimens with immune checkpoint inhibitors (ICPIs).

Future perspectives of TIL therapy

Currently, ACT with TILs is mainly performed with bulk TILs that are hoped to be representative and have the ability to recognize and kill cancer cells throughout the body. Increased knowledge of potential targets, e.g. HPV exposure or neoantigens, for selecting TILs more specifically could increase treatment potential.

Combining ACT with TILs with other anticancer treatment options is also receiving increasing attention.

ICPIs may affect T cells through various pathways. Combining ICPIs with TILs to potentially decrease negative TIL regulation has exciting potential. Another possible combination strategy could be with more classical treatment options such as radiotherapy and/or chemotherapy, which may potentially increase anti-tumour immune responses through different mechanisms.[18,19]

The prognostic impact of the presence of TILs in solid tumours is well known.[20,21] The potential role of TILs as a biomarker should be investigated further in the future to choose who might benefit from this comprehensive treatment regimen.

Conclusion

ACT with TILs is a promising treatment option that has achieved impressive results in metastatic melanoma but is still finding its place in an expanding range of anticancer treatments. Propagation of this treatment option to other malignancies is ongoing and holds great potential. ACT with TILs, however, has its limitations in that it is complex, expensive and still restricted to a few centres worldwide. Furthermore, the current treatment regimens are demanding and only suitable for a small subset of very fit patients. Selection of TILs, methods of predicting who will benefit from the treatment, and combination therapy with other treatment modalities are some of the possible ways of increasing the efficacy of the treatment currently under investigation.

References

1 Kvistborg P, Shu CJ, Heemskerk B, *et al*. TIL therapy broadens the tumor-reactive CD8+ T cell compartment in melanoma patients. *Oncoimmunology* 2012; 1: 409–18.

2 Schumacher TN, Schreiber RD. Neoantigens in cancer immunotherapy. *Science* 2015; 348: 69–74.

3 Schreiber RD. Cancer immunoediting: integrating suppression and promotion. *Science* 2011; 331: 1565–70.

4 Rosenberg SA, Spiess P, Lafreniere R. A new approach to the adoptive immunotherapy of cancer with tumor-infiltrating lymphocytes. *Science* 1986; 233: 1318–21.

5 Topalian SL, Solomon D, Avis FP, *et al*. Immunotherapy of patients with advanced cancer using tumor-infiltrating lymphocytes and recombinant interleukin-2: a pilot study. *J Clin Oncol* 1988; 6: 839–53.

6 Rosenberg SA, Yang JC, Sherry RM, *et al*. Durable complete responses in heavily pretreated patients with metastatic melanoma using T-cell transfer immunotherapy. *Clin Cancer Res* 2011; 17: 4550–7.

7 Besser MJ, Shapira-Frommer R, Schachter J. Tumor-infiltrating lymphocytes: clinical experience. *Cancer J* 2015; 21: 465–9.

8 Geukes Foppen MH, Donia M, Svane IM, Haanen JBAG. Tumor-infiltrating lymphocytes for the treatment of metastatic cancer. *Mol Oncol* 2015; 9: 1918–35.

9 Radvanyi LG. Tumor-infiltrating lymphocyte therapy: addressing prevailing questions. *Cancer J* 2015; 21: 450–64.

10 Dudley ME. Cancer regression and autoimmunity in patients after clonal repopulation with antitumor lymphocytes. *Science* 2002; 298: 850–4.

11 Liao W, Lin J-X, Leonard WJ. Interleukin-2 at the crossroads of effector responses, tolerance, and immunotherapy. *Immunity* 2013; 38: 13–25.

12 Atkins MB, Lotze MT, Dutcher JP, *et al.* High-dose recombinant interleukin 2 therapy for patients with metastatic melanoma: analysis of 270 patients treated between 1985 and 1993. *J Clin Oncol* 1999; 17: 2105–16.

13 Radvanyi LG, Bernatchez C, Zhang M, *et al.* Specific lymphocyte subsets predict response to adoptive cell therapy using expanded autologous tumor-infiltrating lymphocytes in metastatic melanoma patients. *Clin Cancer Res* 2012; 18: 6758–70.

14 Yao X, Ahmadzadeh M, Lu Y-C, *et al.* Levels of peripheral CD4+ FoxP3+ regulatory T cells are negatively associated with clinical response to adoptive immunotherapy of human cancer. *Blood* 2012; 119: 5688–96.

15 Ellebaek E, Iversen TZ, Junker N, *et al.* Adoptive cell therapy with autologous tumor infiltrating lymphocytes and low-dose interleukin-2 in metastatic melanoma patients. *J Transl Med* 2012; 10: 169.

16 Andersen R, Donia M, Ellebaek E, *et al.* Long-lasting complete responses in patients with metastatic melanoma after adoptive cell therapy with tumor-infiltrating lymphocytes and an attenuated IL2 regimen. *Clin Cancer Res* 2016; 22: 3734–45.

17 Stevanović S, Draper LM, Langhan MM, *et al.* Complete regression of metastatic cervical cancer after treatment with human papillomavirus-targeted tumor-infiltrating T cells. *J Clin Oncol* 2015; 33: 1543–50.

18 Wu J, Waxman DJ. Immunogenic chemotherapy: dose and schedule dependence and combination with immunotherapy. *Cancer Lett* 2018; 419: 210–21.

19 Walle T, Martinez Monge R, Cerwenka A, *et al.* Radiation effects on antitumor immune responses: current perspectives and challenges. *Ther Adv Med Oncol* 2018; 10: 1758834017742575.

20 Fridman WH, Pagès F, Sautès-Fridman C, Galon J. The immune contexture in human tumours: impact on clinical outcome. *Nat Rev Cancer* 2012; 12: 298–306.

21 Gooden MJM, de Bock GH, Leffers N, *et al.* The prognostic influence of tumour-infiltrating lymphocytes in cancer: a systematic review with meta-analysis. *Br J Cancer* 2011; 105: 93–103.

01 Cytokine Release Syndrome

Charlotte Graham, Reuben Benjamin

Case history

 A 22-year-old man with relapsed B cell acute lymphoblastic leukaemia (B-ALL) had exhausted all available treatment options, including combination chemotherapy, myeloablative allogenic bone marrow transplant and monoclonal antibody therapy. At the time of his most recent relapse he had isolated bone marrow disease with only 1% B-ALL cells by immunophenotyping, expressing cluster of differentiation (CD) 19, and consistent with minimal residual disease. He was enrolled into a phase I anti-CD19 chimeric antigen receptor (CAR) T cell trial.

He received 5 days of lymphodepleting chemotherapy with fludarabine, cyclophosphamide and alemtuzumab. Bone marrow biopsy following lymphodepletion showed 69% blasts, representing progressive disease. He was then infused with a single dose of anti-CD19 CAR T cells at a total dose of 6×10^6 cells.

Three days after CAR T cell infusion he developed fevers and was empirically treated for febrile neutropenia. Blood cultures showed no bacterial growth. By day 7 he had persistent fevers up to 39°C, and he was tachycardic with a systolic blood pressure of 100 mmHg. He continued to be managed for neutropenic sepsis; supportive measures including intravenous fluids and paracetamol had been deployed in the intervening days. As he was clinically deteriorating and there was no obvious septic source, the working diagnosis was cytokine release syndrome (CRS). The decision was made to give him the interleukin (IL)-6 receptor (IL-6R) antagonist tocilizumab.

Initially, his blood pressure and heart rate normalized, although he continued to spike fevers. By day 9 he was again hypotensive and a second dose of tocilizumab was administered. Despite intravenous fluid resuscitation his systolic blood pressure fell to 80 mmHg; on day 10 he received his third dose of tocilizumab and intravenous corticosteroids. He was transferred to the intensive care unit but stabilized without any requirement for inotropes or other organ support. He was stepped down to the ward a day later prior to being managed in ambulatory care. Expansion of CAR T cells in the blood tracked the clinical course of fevers as did a rise in the cytokines IL-6, interferon (IFN)-γ and IL-10 (Figure 1.1). His bone marrow biopsy on day 14 showed CAR T cells with no evidence of residual B-ALL.

Why did CAR T cell therapy cause CRS in this patient?

What was the aim of treatment for the CRS?

What evidence is there for the use of tocilizumab?

When should corticosteroid therapy be administered?

Can we prevent or ameliorate CRS in patients receiving CAR T cell therapy?

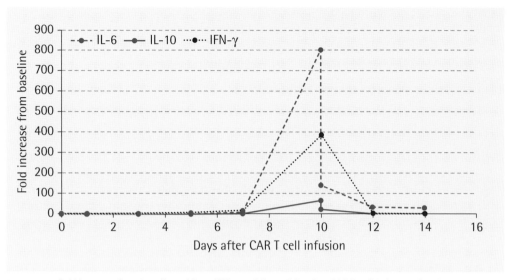

Figure 1.1 Fold increase from baseline of IL-6, IFN-γ and IL-10 following CAR T cell infusion. Cytokines peaked at day 10 when the patient clinically was most unwell from CRS.

Why did CAR T cell therapy cause CRS in this patient?

Anti-CD19 CAR T cells express a single-chain variable fragment of a monoclonal antibody direct-ed against CD19. This is linked to the intracellular signalling domain of the T cell receptor CD3ζ and an additional co-stimulatory domain (4–1BB or CD28). When the CAR T cells were injected into this patient they encountered CD19 expressed on leukaemia cells. Through the artificial CAR construct the T cells received a potent signal, allowing them to kill the leukaemia cells and secrete proinflammatory cytokines. These proinflammatory cytokines cause expansion of the CAR T cells and recruitment of other cells of the immune system such as macrophages. This, however, causes a state of immune overactivation, CRS, with extremely high levels of IL-6, IFN-γ and IL-10. Fever is a marker of CAR T cell expansion and it constitutes grade 1 CRS.[1] If CRS progresses, patients may develop hypotension, coagulopathy and multiorgan dysfunction, which may be fatal.[2] In our patient, the clinical manifestations of CRS coincided with the expansion of CAR T cells in the blood; symptoms resolved once the leukaemia cells were cleared and the CAR T cells were no longer coming into contact with CD19. Patients with a higher disease burden are at greater risk of severe CRS,[3] and by the time of infusion our patient had developed bulky bone marrow disease.

What was the aim of treatment for the CRS?

CRS may be catastrophic. Patients may become hypoxic with acute respiratory distress syndrome requiring ventilatory support. Liver and renal failure may develop. Cardiac dysfunction may also occur, which is thought to be stress-induced cardiomyopathy similar to Takotsubo.[2] CRS is also a sign, however, that CAR T cell therapy is performing its anti-leukaemia function. The focus of CRS-directed therapy in our patient was to prevent end-organ dysfunction without disabling the CAR T cells. Supportive care, with meticulous attention to fluid balance and blood pressure in the intensive care unit, may help bring patients though CRS safely. IL-6, a cytokine secreted by T cells, monocytes and macrophages, may be markedly elevated in patients with CRS. It is a proinflammatory cytokine thought to play a role in the organ dysfunction seen. Unlike IFN-γ, it is not directly involved in T cell cytotoxic function and therefore may be targeted without blocking CAR T cells. IL-6R blockade is one targeted approach for CRS, with the majority of clinical data available for tocilizumab, which is why it was used first line.[4]

What evidence is there for the use of tocilizumab?

Tocilizumab is an IL-6R antagonist. It is the first US Food and Drug Administration (FDA) licensed therapy for the treatment of severe CRS. Licensing was granted based on pooled data from a retrospective analysis of a number of clinical trials in which tocilizumab was used for severe or life-threatening CRS, finding that 69% of patients recovered within 2 weeks.[5]

IL-6 may cause activation of the Janus kinase–signal transducers and activators of transcription (JAK-STAT) pathway by two methods: cytokine-inducible SH2-containing protein (CIS) signalling by IL-6 binding to the membrane-bound IL-6R, which occurs at low concentrations; or, when the soluble IL-6R binds IL-6, which occurs at high concentrations, it is able to signal via membrane-bound glycoprotein (gp) 130. These two different signalling pathways are important, as they broaden the number of tissues IL-6 can affect. IL-6R is only expressed on haematopoietic cells, whereas gp130 is expressed on most tissues and explains the wide-ranging deleterious effect of CRS.[4] As tocilizumab binds to the IL-6R it blocks both pathways by which IL-6 can signal during CRS.

When should corticosteroid therapy be administered?

Corticosteroids have a more global effect on cytokine secretion by T cells and are known to reduce normal T cell proliferation and activation. There is a reluctance to use corticosteroids in patients who have received CAR T cell therapy in case they impede the anti-leukaemia activity of the adoptive cells. At very high doses (>100 mg prednisolone), steroids have led to the loss of CAR T cells.[3] Despite this, a growing number of groups are using corticosteroids with a short half-life in cases of life-threatening CRS, without seeing a negative impact on T cell expansion.[2] It may be that by the time CRS has developed, adequate CAR T cell expansion and activation have occurred, allowing clearance of leukaemia cells, as happened in our patient. Current guidelines recommend corticosteroids in patients with persistent CRS following IL-6R-blocking therapy or in those who are developing signs of end-organ dysfunction.[4]

Neurotoxicity is another side effect that may be seen with anti-CD19 CAR T cell therapy. It may develop with CRS, or independently of it. In patients with neurotoxicity, corticosteroids are preferred as they treat both conditions.[6] There is a trend to avoid tocilizumab if neurotoxicity is present, as it increases serum-free levels of IL-6 (potentially allowing more IL-6 to cross the blood–brain barrier),[4] but currently there is limited understanding of the pathophysiology of neurotoxicity and how best to manage it.

Can we prevent or ameliorate CRS in patients receiving CAR T cell therapy?

To ensure optimal management of CRS, patients should be admitted to a ward with nursing and medical staff educated and experienced in monitoring for the complications of CAR T cell therapy. The intensive care unit supporting CAR T cell patients should similarly have expertise in managing CRS and must be notified of the timing of cell infusion and provide close liaison with an outreach team.

CAR T cell infusion should be delayed or cancelled in patients with active infection or developing organ dysfunction, as both increase the likelihood of a fatal outcome. Where possible, disease bulk should be controlled prior to infusion.

Once CAR T cell therapy has been administered, patients must be monitored closely with daily weights, fluid balance chart, ECG/cardiac monitoring and daily bloods including C-reactive protein (CRP) and ferritin.[4] If available, serum cytokine measurements may provide further information. Early CRS is clinically indistinguishable from febrile neutropenia and as most patients will be neutropenic from lymphodepletion, infection should be screened for and treated as per local neutropenic sepsis guidelines. Granulocyte colony-stimulating factor (GCSF) may be administered to shorten the period of neutropenia.[4]

There should be a low threshold for initiating CRS-specific therapy with tocilizumab in patients with hypotension not responding to intravenous fluids or who are not improving with supportive therapy alone. Patients should be transferred to the intensive care unit for closer monitoring if their condition does not improve.

Conclusion and learning points

- CRS is a common and expected side effect of CAR T cell therapy.
- The clinical condition of the patient may rapidly deteriorate, with life-threatening complications.
- Treatment with the IL-6R blocker tocilizumab is the first FDA-approved treatment for severe CRS.
- Corticosteroids should be used in patients not responding to tocilizumab and in those developing end-organ dysfunction.
- The intensive care team is vital to the delivery of CAR T cell therapy.

References

1 Lee DW, Gardner R, Porter DL, *et al*. Current concepts in the diagnosis and management of cytokine release syndrome. *Blood* 2014; 124: 188–95.

2 Maude SL, Barrett D, Teachey DT, *et al*. Managing cytokine release syndrome associated with novel T cell-engaging therapies. *Cancer J* 2014; 20: 119–22.

3 Davila ML, Riviere I, Wang X, *et al*. Efficacy and toxicity management of 19–28z CAR T cell therapy in B cell acute lymphoblastic leukemia. *Sci Transl Med* 2014; 6: 224ra25.

4 Neelapu SS, Tummala S, Kebriaei P, *et al*. Chimeric antigen receptor T-cell therapy – assessment and management of toxicities. *Nat Rev Clin Oncol* 2018; 15: 47–62.

5 US Food and Drug Administration (2017). *FDA approves tisagenlecleucel for B-cell ALL and tocilizumab for cytokine release syndrome*. Available from: www.fda.gov/drugs/informationondrugs/approveddrugs/ucm574154.htm (accessed 26 February 2018).

6 Gardener R, Leger KJ, Annesley CE, *et al*. Decreased rates of severe CRS seen with early intervention strategies for CD19 CAR-T cell toxicity management. Presented at: American Society of Haematology Annual Meeting, San Diego, CA, USA, December 2016. Abstract 586.

Further reading

- Bonifant CL, Jackson HJ, Brentjens RJ, Curran KJ. Toxicity and management in CAR T-cell therapy. *Mol Ther Oncolytics* 2016; 3: 16011.

02 High-Dose Interleukin-2-Induced Myocarditis

Manon Pillai, Fiona Thistlethwaite

Case history

A 55-year-old woman presented with small volume metastatic disease 2 years after radical nephrectomy for a T3 clear cell renal cell carcinoma (RCC). At first oncological assessment she was of good performance status with no significant medical co-morbidities and was deemed suitable for first line treatment with high-dose inter-leukin-2 (HD IL-2) therapy.

She was admitted for the first cycle of treatment and completed 19 doses of HD IL-2. Reassessment CT imaging at 3 months revealed a partial response to treat-ment and she was readmitted for a second course of eight doses, without compli-cations. She developed central chest pain at rest 24 h after her final dose. Although her ECG revealed no acute abnormality, troponin I was elevated at 0.25 µg/l (<0.017 µg/l). She was assessed by the cardiology team and both echocardiography and coronary angiography were normal. Her troponin I normalized over 48 h and she experienced no further chest pain. No clear causes for these symptoms were identified.

She started a third cycle of HD IL-2 therapy, as her symptoms had resolved, cardiac investigations were normal and CT imaging at 6 months revealed an ongoing excellent response to treatment with almost complete resolution of her metastatic disease. Again, this was initially well tolerated and she completed eight doses. After her ninth dose, however, she developed dysarthria and left-sided facial droop. Intracranial imaging revealed an area of abnormality in the right hemisphere consistent with an embolic infarct. Investigations revealed elevated troponin I. New T wave inversion on ECG and transthoracic echo confirmed a left atrial thrombus with impaired left ventricular systolic function. She was commenced on therapeutic anticoagulation. Cardiac magnetic resonance (CMR) imaging with late gadolinium enhancement revealed non-ischaemic mid-wall late enhancement in keeping with acute oedema caused by myocarditis. Other causes of myocarditis were excluded and a diagnosis of HD IL-2-induced myocarditis was made. Medical therapy with beta-blockade was commenced.

Over the next 48 h her neurological symptoms completely resolved. Repeat echocar-diography 3 months after the acute event revealed resolution of the atrial thrombus, and a repeat CMR demonstrated normally enhancing myocardium with restoration of systolic function. Cardiac medications were subsequently stopped. CT imaging over

4 years after completion of HD IL-2 therapy confirmed ongoing sustained response. She remains under active surveillance.

What is the current evidence for the use of HD IL-2 in the management of metastatic RCC?

How is HD IL-2 administered?

What are the frequent toxicities of HD IL-2?

How is treatment-induced myocarditis diagnosed and treated?

In this era of targeted immunotherapies, is there a continued role for HD IL-2 in the future management of RCC?

What is the current evidence for the use of HD IL-2 in the management of metastatic RCC?

Cytokines play an integral role in immune biology, and attempts have been made to harness their potential as anticancer therapies. IL-2 has a wide range of effects on a variety of immune cells, and T lymphocytes in particular, where it aids in the propagation and differentiation of effector T cells.[1] Clinical application of IL-2 has been studied in a variety of immunogenic tumours. In 1989, Rosenberg *et al.*[2] reported a response rate to HD IL-2 treatment of 22% and 24% in patients with RCC and melanoma, respectively, with 7% of RCC patients achieving a durable complete response.

Careful selection of RCC patients based on baseline histopathological biomarkers has improved responses, with overall response rates reaching 43% and complete response rates 21% in one UK centre.[3] The same group demonstrated that patients with fewer sites of disease (one or two involved organs) and those completing a high number of doses with their first cycle of HD IL-2 (over 16 doses) were more likely to derive therapeutic benefit.

HD IL-2 is usually considered as a first line treatment but may also safely be administered following standard targeted small molecule therapy, where response rates and toxicities are comparable to those of untreated patients.[4]

Efforts have been made to decrease the potential toxicities associated with HD IL-2 by altering the administered dose. This is associated, however, with decreased efficacy and a lower proportion of complete responders.[5] High-dose treatment therefore remains the standard of care. In view of the consistent, durable response rates seen, HD IL-2 remains a valid option in the management of highly selected patients with advanced RCC.

How is HD IL-2 administered?

Currently, HD IL-2 is delivered at one specialist cancer centre in the UK (The Christie NHS Foundation Trust). Patients considered for treatment are medically fit, with a good performance status and minimal other comorbidities. All patients must have undergone a prior nephrectomy. Treatment is delivered in 12 weekly cycles with the patient admitted at week 1 and week 3. During these inpatient weeks, HD IL-2 is administered intravenously every 8 h for a total of 5 days. Supportive medications are administered concomitantly. Reassessment CT imaging is conducted at week 11 and if a radiological response is seen and the treatment has been tolerated well, a further cycle is administered. Treatment will continue every 12 weeks until a complete or best response is achieved.

What are the frequent toxicities of HD IL-2?

Treatment with HD IL-2 may be complicated by significant toxicities. Anticipating and proactively managing toxicities are key to successful treatment delivery. Immediate toxicities are common and are frequently a result of capillary leak syndrome, which develops secondary to the release of HD IL-2-induced circulating cytokines and subsequent activation of complement products, neutrophils and endothelial cell antigens.[6] Activated cytokines increase capillary permeability and lower vascular resistance, leading to fluid shifting from the bloodstream to the extravascular space and the development of hypovolaemia, tachycardia, weight gain and pulmonary oedema. Hyperpyrexia, rigors and flu-like symptoms are also frequently seen as a direct effect of cytokine release. These acute toxicities are managed supportively but aggressively, with intravenous fluids, antipyretics and antibiotics as needed. Antihypertensive agents are discontinued prior to commencing treatment and critical care medical teams should be alerted if patients do not respond to supportive treatments.

Prolonged or severe hypovolaemia may also lead to end-organ damage; therefore, renal, hepatic, bowel, cardiac and cognitive function must be closely monitored during treatment. Key organ function may also be further compounded by HD IL-2-induced lymphoid infiltration leading to local inflammation. Significant impairment of organ function should lead to discontinuation of treatment.

The half-life of HD IL-2 is measured in minutes; therefore, the majority of toxicities resolve rapidly and completely on treatment discontinuation. Endocrine (frequently affecting the thyroid gland) and dermatological toxicities, however, may develop up to 6 weeks after treatment. In contrast to immediate toxicities, thyroid abnormalities are frequently non-reversible and patients need lifelong replacement therapy.

How is treatment-induced myocarditis diagnosed and treated?

While HD IL-2 administration may lead to a broad range of cardiac toxicities, and hypotension secondary to hypovolaemia is very frequently seen, other more significant cardiac complications are rare. Supraventricular tachyarrhythmias, which are usually brief and self limiting, may occur but do not regularly alter management.

Myocarditis is reported in up to 5% of patients and occurs secondary to IL-2-induced cytokine-driven endothelial cell damage.[7] Although it is a recognized complication of HD IL-2, myocarditis may pose a diagnostic challenge to treating oncologists as its clinical presentation may be variable and as a result the diagnosis may be missed. The presentation of the patient in this case with an embolic intracranial event is very rare. The range of clinical symptoms associated with myocarditis may be broad and extends from no symptoms with incidental elevated cardiac enzymes to cardiac arrhythmias, ischaemic ECG changes and chest pain. Obtaining a definitive diagnosis is therefore difficult.

Prompt diagnosis and initiation of management once the diagnosis is made are essential and may prevent long-term consequences. When myocarditis is suspected, serial ECGs should be conducted with paired serum cardiac enzymes. Echocardiography may be helpful in evaluating ventricular function but may lack specificity and demonstrates limited ability to characterize the underlying myocardium. As the main differential diagnosis is an acute coronary syndrome, early involvement of cardiology teams is strongly advised and coronary artery angiography may also be appropriate to exclude an ischaemic event. CMR imaging has recently emerged as the new gold standard for diagnosis of myocarditis and has the advantage of being both non-invasive and able to differentiate between different aetiologies of chest pain and elevated cardiac enzymes. It has proven effective in the diagnosis of IL-2-induced myocarditis in a number of case reports[7,8] and should be considered in every case.

Management of HD IL-2-induced myocarditis is again supportive and should be directed by specialist cardiology teams. IL-2 treatment should be withheld, potentially permanently. In the majority of cases myocarditis is fully reversible and cardiac function returns to baseline with time. Further HD IL-2 treatment may be discussed with the patient following a frank examination of the potential benefits and risks of further toxicity.

To reduce the incidence of myocarditis it is imperative prior to treatment to identify patients who are at higher risk of developing it. Pretreatment cardiac evaluation, including routine ECG and stress echocardiogram for older patients or those with any pre-existing cardiac condition, should be strongly considered.

In this era of targeted immunotherapies, is there a continued role for HD IL-2 in the future management of RCC?

Recent developments in the field of immunotherapy, and the approval of several immune check-point inhibitors (ICPIs) in particular, have transformed the management of several cancers. The anti-programmed cell death protein 1 (PD-1) monoclonal antibody nivolumab is approved in RCC following the failure of first line targeted therapies, where it demonstrates superior response rates and overall survival when compared with everolimus.[9] The combination of the anti-cytotoxic T lymphocyte-associated protein 4 (CTLA-4) monoclonal antibody ipilimumab with nivolumab has also recently demonstrated superiority when compared with sunitinib in intermediate- and poor-risk RCC patients[10] and will likely achieve regulatory approval in this setting in the near future. There is also growing interest in combining ICPIs with small molecules; the preliminary data from the Avelumab in Combination with Axitinib in Advanced Renal Cell Cancer (JAVELIN Renal 100) clinical trial in previously untreated patients suggest that this approach is safe, with encouraging anti-tumour activity.[11]

ICPI-related complications are well documented, particularly when these agents are administered in combination. They carry a more favourable toxicity profile, however, compared with HD IL-2, and their administration and treatment schedules are more acceptable to both patients and treating physicians. As the data surrounding the efficacy of ICPI therapy in RCC mature, it seems likely that these agents will replace HD IL-2 in the treatment of RCC in the future.

While the role of HD IL-2 in the management of RCC may be diminishing, the complete response rates seen with this therapy in carefully preselected patients remain impressive. Novel work is attempting to exploit this by developing a more tolerable form of IL-2 that may be associated with less systemic toxicity. Early phase studies of an immune cytokine consisting of a variant form of IL-2 linked to a monoclonal antibody directed against fibroblast activation protein-α in a variety of solid malignancies is ongoing and a further study of this agent in combination with programmed death-ligand 1 (PD-L1) and vascular endothelial growth factor (VEGF)-directed monoclonal antibodies in RCC patients is currently recruiting (Study to Evaluate Safety, Pharmacokinetics and Therapeutic Activity of RO6874281 as a Combination Therapy in Participants with Unresectable Advanced and/or Metastatic RCC).

Conclusion and learning points

- HD IL-2 can produce impressive, durable complete response rates in carefully selected patients with metastatic clear cell RCC.

- HD IL-2 treatment may be toxic. Anticipating and proactively managing toxicities are key to successful treatment delivery.

- Patients should be screened prior to treatment and evaluated for cardiovascular complications. Only patients with suitable performance status and minimal comorbidities should receive treatment.

- Myocarditis occurs in up to 5% of patients and is completely reversible in the vast majority.

- Prompt treatment and involvement of specialist cardiology teams are key to preventing long-term complications.

- The development of variant forms of IL-2 may decrease its toxicity profile and widen its administration to different patients and immunogenic cancer types.

References

1 Boyman O, Sprent J. The role of interleukin-2 during homeostasis and activation of the immune system. *Nat Rev Immunol* 2012; 12: 180–90.

2 Rosenberg SA, Lotze MT, Yang YC, *et al.* Experience with the use of high-dose interleukin-2 in the treatment of 652 cancer patients. *Ann Surg* 1989; 210: 474–84; discussion 484–5.

3 Chow S, Galvis V, Pillai M, *et al.* High-dose interleukin2 – a 10-year single-site experience in the treatment of metastatic renal cell carcinoma: careful selection of patients gives an excellent outcome. *J Immunother Cancer* 2016; 4: 67.

4 Evans M, Chow S, Galvis V, *et al.* Evaluating the place of IL-2 in the management of metastatic renal cell carcinoma in the era of targeted therapy. Presented at: ESMO symposium on immuno-oncology, Geneva, 21–22 November 2014.

5 Yang JC, Sherry RM, Steinberg SM, *et al.* Randomized study of high-dose and low-dose interleukin-2 in patients with metastatic renal cancer. *J Clin Oncol* 2003; 21: 3127–32.

6 Schwartz RN, Stover L, Dutcher JP. Managing toxicities of high-dose interleukin-2. *Oncology (Williston Park)* 2002; 16 (11 suppl 13): 11–20.

7 Chow S, Cove-Smith L, Schmitt M, Hawkins R. High-dose interleukin 2-induced myocarditis: can myocardial damage reversibility be assessed by cardiac MRI? *J Immunother* 2014; 37: 304–8.

8 Tan MC, Ortega-Legaspi JM, Cheng SF, *et al.* Acute myocarditis following high-dose interleukin-2 treatment. *J Cardiol Cases* 2017; 15: 28–31.

9 Motzer RJ, Escudier B, McDermott DF, *et al.* Nivolumab versus everolimus in advanced renal-cell carcinoma. *N Engl J Med* 2015; 373: 1803–13.

10 Motzer RJ, Tannir NM, McDermott DF, *et al.* Nivolumab plus ipilimumab versus sunitinib in advanced renal-cell carcinoma. *N Engl J Med* 2018; 378: 1277–90.

11 Choueiri TK, Larkin J, Oya M, *et al.* Preliminary results for avelumab plus axitinib as first-line therapy in patients with advanced clear-cell renal-cell carcinoma (JAVELIN Renal 100): an open-label, dose-finding and dose-expansion, phase 1b trial. *Lancet Oncol* 2018; 19: 451–60.

03 Multiorgan Toxicity after Combination Immunotherapy in Melanoma

Jennifer Thomas, Lewis Au, James Larkin

Case history

A 78-year-old woman underwent wide local excision for an isolated 25 mm thickness *BRAF/NRAS/KIT* wild-type neurotropic cutaneous melanoma on her right cheek, followed by adjuvant radiotherapy given a positive resection margin. Her medical history was significant only for depression, for which she took citalopram. Twelve months after her initial diagnosis a surveillance PET-CT scan demonstrated new bone and liver metastases, and she commenced systemic therapy with the combination of ipilimumab and nivolumab. This was complicated by subclinical thyroiditis and subsequent hypothyroidism, which was managed with oral levothyroxine replacement. A follow-up PET-CT scan after four cycles showed complete metabolic response after 6 months of treatment and she went on to continue 2 weekly maintenance nivolumab.

Nine months after commencing treatment, she presented to A&E with nausea, vomiting and chest heaviness. ECGs showed sinus rhythm with deep T wave inversion in precordial leads V1–V4. There were no conduction abnormalities. Troponin I was elevated at 0.053 µg/l (upper limit of normal [ULN] 0.04 µg/l), with brain natriuretic peptide (BNP) at 437.5 ng/l (ULN 25 ng/l). A bedside echocardiogram showed mild apical hypokinesia. On the advice of cardiology she commenced regular aspirin, with a plan for urgent cardiac MRI and to start intravenous methylprednisolone in the event of further ECG changes, rising troponin I level or clinical deterioration.

At 48 h from admission, ECGs remained stable and troponin I was falling. She developed severe, bloody diarrhoea, however, and was commenced on intravenous methylprednisolone at a dose of 2 mg/kg per day. Cardiac MRI on day 4 confirmed myocardial oedema and inflammation in the apical segments, mid-septum and mid-anterior wall, with no myocardial infarction, infiltration or fibrosis. Appearances were reported as in keeping with acute myocarditis. By day 5, diarrhoea had started to resolve and methylprednisolone was reduced to 1 mg/kg per day. Steroid dosing was further reduced, titrating to ongoing clinical improvement. Oral ramipril was added and titrated to blood pressure.

On day 9, she developed grade 1 hepatitis with alanine aminotransferase (ALT) 1.24 µkat/l (ULN 0.68 µkat/l). This progressively worsened over the next 3 days, peaking at ALT 1.87 µkat/l (grade 2). In view of her evolving, multiorgan toxicities, intravenous methylprednisolone was escalated to 500 mg/kg per day and oral mycophenolate mofetil was added at a dose of 1 g twice daily. Liver ultrasound was unremarkable and a liver screen did not reveal an infective cause for her elevated ALT.

By day 20, ALT and troponin I were falling, diarrhoea had resolved, and repeat cardiac MRI showed partial resolution of myocardial oedema. Steroids were gradually withdrawn without further complications and she has since remained clinically well. Nivolumab was permanently discontinued; nevertheless, subsequent restaging imaging demonstrated a maintained complete response.

What is the evidence base for the use of combination immunotherapy in advanced melanoma?

What is the incidence of toxicity associated with this regimen? What are the key principles guiding management?

How does immune checkpoint inhibitor (ICPI)-related cardiotoxicity manifest?

How should you approach work-up and management of a patient with suspected myocarditis on immunotherapy?

How is management affected by the presence of multiple toxicities?

What is the evidence base for the use of combination immunotherapy in advanced melanoma?

CheckMate 067 was a landmark study informing the use of combination treatment with the ICPIs nivolumab (anti-programmed cell death protein 1 [PD-1]) plus ipilimumab (anti-cytotoxic T lymphocyte-associated protein 4 [CTLA-4]) as first line therapy for advanced melanoma.[1,2] It followed studies that demonstrated clinical efficacy of anti-CTLA-4[3,4] and anti-PD-1[5-7] agents as monotherapies for the treatment of metastatic melanoma. In this international, multicentre, double-blind phase III trial, 945 patients with previously untreated stage IV or unresectable stage III melanoma were randomized 1:1:1 to receive nivolumab alone (3 mg/kg every 2 weeks; n=316), ipilimumab alone (3 mg/kg every 3 weeks in four doses; n=315), or the two in combination (1 mg/kg nivolumab plus 3 mg/kg ipilimumab every 3 weeks in four doses, followed by 3 mg/kg nivolumab every 2 weeks; n=314). While the study was not powered to detect differences between the combination and nivolumab arms, overall survival (OS), progression-free survival (PFS) and overall response rates all favoured combination therapy numerically. The OS rates at 3 years were 58%, 52% and 34% for combination therapy, nivolumab alone and ipilimumab alone, respectively. At a minimum follow-up of 28 months, median PFS was 11.5 months vs 6.9 months for the combination arm compared with nivolumab alone (HR 0.78; 95% CI 0.64, 0.96), and overall response rates were 58% vs 44% also favouring combination treatment.

For the subset of patients with *BRAF*-mutant melanoma (around 40%), mitogen-activated protein kinase (MAPK) pathway-targeted therapy with serine/threonine-protein kinase B-Raf (BRAF) and mitogen-activated protein kinase kinase (MEK) inhibitors offers another avenue of treatment for advanced disease. To date there are no randomized, prospective studies directly comparing immunotherapy with targeted therapy in this setting.

What is the incidence of toxicity associated with this regimen? What are the key principles guiding management?

Combination therapy is associated with a higher incidence of immune-related adverse events (irAEs) than either agent alone. irAEs may affect almost any organ, but the most commonly described are skin (affecting 59.1% in the combination cohort), gastrointestinal (46.3%), hepatic

(30%), endocrine (30%) and pulmonary (7%).[1] In CheckMate 067, grade 3 or 4 toxicity was reported in 59% of the combination group, compared with 21% and 28% in the nivolumab and ipilimumab arms, respectively. This prompted permanent treatment discontinuation for 39.3% of patients in the combination cohort.[1,2]

Effective management of severe (grade 3 or 4) toxicity depends on prompt recognition and early initiation of systemic glucocorticoids, often required at high doses of intravenous methylprednisolone 1–2 mg/kg per day. If this does not lead to rapid improvement, consideration should be given to the addition of other immunomodulatory agents such as infliximab or mycophenolate mofetil.[8] Importantly, the outcomes for patients who require immunosuppression and/or discontinue immunotherapy early for toxicity do not appear to be compromised compared with those who do not experience severe irAEs. This was explored in a pooled analysis of patients receiving ipilimumab and nivolumab as part of CheckMate 067 or CheckMate 069 (phase II), where there were no differences between those with and those without severe irAEs in overall response rate (58% vs 50%) and median PFS (8.4 vs 10.8 months [HR 0.99; 95% CI 0.72, 1.37; $p=0.966$]). Median OS was not reached in either group (HR 0.79; 95% CI 0.55, 1.17; $p=0.2344$).[9] Immunosuppressive therapies should therefore not be unduly withheld for treatment of severe irAEs. Consideration of further ICPI treatment after resolution of toxicity requires careful analysis of the risks and benefits, and would rarely be considered after any grade 4 events. Endocrine toxicity is an exception: gland function is unlikely to recover and those affected require lifelong hormone replacement.[1,2] ICPI treatment may usually be safely continued once patients are asymptomatic and stable on appropriate replacement therapy.

How does ICPI–related cardiotoxicity manifest?

Immune-mediated cardiac toxicity is a rare but serious complication of ICPIs. Pharmacovigilance data of 20,594 patients treated with ipilimumab, nivolumab, or both, report severe myocarditis in 0.09%, rising to 0.27% among those who received the two agents in combination.[10] In addition to myocarditis there have been case reports of myocardial fibrosis, pericarditis, heart block and Takotsubo-like cardiomyopathy. In a case series of eight patients with cardiac toxicity following ICPIs, it was fatal in three despite maximal immunosuppressive therapy.[11]

Some insight into the pathogenesis of cardiac toxicity comes from a detailed study of two cases of fatal fulminant myocarditis in patients treated with combination ipilimumab and nivolumab.[8] Both patients presented with ECG changes (conduction delay or ST segment abnormalities) and elevated troponin I, with or without chest pain. Echocardiography demonstrated preserved left ventricular ejection fractions. In both cases conduction disturbances persisted despite prompt intravenous glucocorticoids and both fell into refractory arrhythmias with unsuccessful resuscitation attempts. Postmortem histological analysis demonstrated lymphocytic infiltration of the myocardium and SA and AV nodes. Of note, programmed death-ligand 1 (PD-L1) was expressed on the injured myocardium and infiltrating cluster of differentiation (CD) 8+ T cells. T cell receptor sequencing from CD8+ cells infiltrating patients' myocardium, skeletal muscle and tumour samples revealed commonality of expanded T cell clones, suggesting possible recognition of shared antigens between these tissues.

How should you approach work–up and management of a patient with suspected myocarditis on immunotherapy?

Clinicians should have a high index of suspicion for immune-mediated toxicity in any patient who presents with cardiac symptoms such as chest pain, dyspnoea or palpitations. Initial work-up should include serial ECGs, troponin I and BNP measurement and echocardiography. Currently, cardiac MRI is the most sensitive imaging modality for detection of inflammatory changes, but treatment should not be delayed while awaiting investigations where there is strong clinical suspicion of immune-mediated pathology. Specialist cardiology input should be sought early and, given the propensity towards development of arrhythmias, cardiac monitoring is advisable if there is evidence of ECG changes.

To date there is no high-level evidence to direct specific management of cardiac toxicity. High-dose intravenous methylprednisolone is the mainstay of treatment. Given that pathological examination in the cases above was similar to that seen in acute allograft rejection, it has been postulated that anti-thymocyte globulin may also be of benefit.[10] Anti-tumour necrosis factor (TNF) therapy, mycophenolate mofetil or tacrolimus could also be considered in refractory cases.[8]

How is management affected by the presence of multiple toxicities?

It is not uncommon for patients treated with combination ICPIs to develop toxicity affecting multiple organs, either concurrently or in sequence. In a pooled retrospective study of 409 patients who received combination immunotherapy, half of those who discontinued treatment early because of irAEs had toxicity affecting more than one organ.[9] Kinetics of specific irAEs vary, but a large proportion of toxicities emerge in the induction phase (i.e. the first four cycles) of combination treatment.[8]

Multidisciplinary involvement in such cases is beneficial, particularly where the management of toxicity affecting one organ may impact on another; one example would be in patients with ICPI-induced pancreatic endocrine deficiency whose blood sugar control may be affected by high-dose steroids. Additional consideration should be given to drug absorption, metabolism and interactions in the context of impaired organ function. Vigilance is required during steroid weaning, as new irAEs may be 'unmasked' on reducing doses of steroids commenced for the first event.

Patients with multiorgan toxicity may require long courses of high-dose systemic glucocorticoids; care should be taken to minimize the associated risk of opportunistic infection with *Pneumocystis jirovecii* pneumonia (PJP), and consideration given to proximal myopathy effects, gastrointestinal side effects, impact on mood, and bone health.

Conclusion and learning points

- Ipilimumab/nivolumab combination immunotherapy is an effective treatment for advanced melanoma.
- Combination immunotherapy is associated with a higher incidence of irAEs than either agent given alone. Most toxicities resolve with steroids and, where necessary, discontinuation of immunotherapy because of severe toxicity is not associated with worse outcomes.
- Immune-mediated cardiac toxicity is a rare but serious complication of ICPI therapy. It may follow a fulminant course and should be suspected in any patient presenting with cardiac signs or symptoms.
- Suspected cardiac toxicity should be managed with high-dose intravenous methylprednisolone and requires close communication with experienced cardiology centres.
- Multiorgan immune toxicity is not uncommon and may pose additional challenges. Where steroids are required at immunosuppressive doses for >1 month, PJP prophylaxis is recommended.

References

1 Larkin J, Chiarion-Sileni V, González R, *et al.* Combined nivolumab and ipilimumab or monotherapy in untreated melanoma. *N Engl J Med* 2015; 373: 23–34.

2 Wolchok J, Chiarion-Sileni V, González R, *et al.* Overall survival with combined nivolumab and ipilimumab in advanced melanoma. *N Engl J Med* 2017; 377: 1345–56.

3 Hodi FS, O'Day SJ, McDermott DF, *et al.* Improved survival with ipilimumab in patients with metastatic melanoma. *N Engl J Med* 2010; 363: 711–23.

4 Robert C, Thomas L, Bondarenko I, *et al.* Ipilimumab plus dacarbazine for previously untreated metastatic melanoma. *N Engl J Med* 2011; 364: 2517–26.

5 Weber JS, D'Angelo SP, Minor D, *et al.* Nivolumab versus chemotherapy in patients with advanced melanoma who progressed after anti-CTLA-4 treatment (CheckMate 037): a randomised, controlled, open-label, phase 3 trial. *Lancet Oncol* 2015; 16: 375–84.

6 Robert C, Long G, Brady B, *et al.* Nivolumab in previously untreated melanoma without *BRAF* mutation. *N Engl J Med* 2015; 372: 320–30.

7 Robert C, Schachter J, Long G, *et al.* Pembrolizumab versus ipilimumab in advanced melanoma. *N Engl J Med* 2015; 372: 2521–32.

8 Haanen JBAG, Carbonnel F, Robert C, *et al.* Management of toxicities from immunotherapy: ESMO clinical practice guidelines for diagnosis, treatment and follow-up. *Ann Oncol* 2017; 28 (suppl 4): iv119–42.

9 Schadendorf D, Wolchok J, Hodi S, *et al.* Efficacy and safety outcomes for patients with advanced melanoma who discontinued treatment with nivolumab and ipilimumab because of adverse events; a pooled analysis of randomized phase II and phase III trials. *J Clin Oncol* 2017; 35: 3807–14.

10 Johnson D, Balko J, Compton M, *et al.* Fulminant myocarditis with combination immune checkpoint blockade. *N Engl J Med* 2016; 375: 1749–55.

11 Heinzerling L, Ott PA, Hodi FS, *et al.* Cardiotoxicity associated with CTLA4 and PD1 blocking immunotherapy. *J Immunother Cancer* 2016; 4: 50.

Further reading

• Postow M, Sidlow R, Hellmann M, *et al.* Immune-related adverse events associated with immune checkpoint blockade. *N Engl J Med* 2018; 378: 158–68.

• Spain L, Diem S, Larkin J. Management of toxicities of immune checkpoint inhibitors. *Cancer Treat Rev* 2016; 44: 51–60.

04 Immune-Related Endocrine Toxicity after Immune Checkpoint Inhibitor Therapy

Alec Paschalis, Matthew Wheater

Case history

A 60-year-old man with a history of a 4.7 mm (pT4) *BRAF* wild-type malignant mela-noma of the right arm, previously treated with wide local excision and right axillary lymph node dissection, presented with multiple new subcutaneous deposits over the medial aspect of his right forearm. His only other medical history was of hyperten-sion, and his performance status was zero. Staging CT confirmed metastatic disease with recurrence in the right axilla as well as multiple new subcutaneous deposits in his abdominal wall. He was therefore commenced on systemic therapy with ipili-mumab. In spite of this, after three cycles of treatment his skin lesions continued to progress; therefore, his treatment was switched to pembrolizumab. While clinically this led to an improvement in his melanocytic deposits, following his third dose of treatment he presented with severe fatigue and abdominal pain.

On examination he was hypotensive but remained apyrexial with a soft and non-tender abdomen and normal bowel sounds. Initial investigations revealed hyponatraemia (121 mmol/l) and undetectable cortisol levels.

Clinically he appeared in Addisonian crisis and was resuscitated with intravenous fluids and hydrocortisone. His immunotherapy was held and further investigations were performed (Table 4.1) including a short Synacthen test and serum adrenocor-ticotropic hormone (ACTH) that were indicative of secondary adrenal insufficiency. A restaging CT scan showed a positive response to treatment and no evidence of adrenal metastases; brain MRI was normal. Taken together these results indicated a diagnosis of secondary adrenal insufficiency as a result of acute hypophysitis, most likely caused by ipilimumab.

Over the next 5 days the patient's symptoms improved with steroid replacement therapy, and his blood pressure, serum sodium and morning cortisol levels all nor-malized. Subsequently he was converted to an oral steroid maintenance regimen of 10 mg hydrocortisone in the morning, 10 mg at lunch and 5 mg in the evening and discharged home following endocrinology review and formal steroid education.

He was seen back in the oncology clinic a week later, where he was recommenced on pembrolizumab, to which he has had a complete response. He continues on steroid replacement therapy.

Table 4.1 Summary of investigations performed.

Test	Result	Normal range
Serum osmolality, mmol/kg	253	275–295
Urine osmolality, mmol/kg	394	300–800
Random urine sodium, mmol/l	14	NA
Short Synacthen test (cortisol 30 min post-Synacthen), nmol/l	549	NA[a]
ACTH, pmol/l	<5	0–46
CT chest/abdomen/pelvis	Positive response to treatment with significant decrease in size of right axillary soft tissue mass and anterior abdominal wall subcutaneous nodules No evidence of adrenal metastases	
MRI pituitary	Pituitary gland of normal size with a concave superior margin Pituitary stalk of normal appearance No evidence of hypophysitis or intracranial metastases	

[a]Normal response corresponds with plasma cortisol ≥420 nmol/l after 30 min.

How common are endocrine toxicities and how may they be identified?

What is hypophysitis and what symptoms does it cause?

How is hypophysitis diagnosed?

What information would you provide to this patient on discharge?

How would you manage this patient's subsequent anticancer therapy?

How common are endocrine toxicities and how may they be identified?

The true incidence of immune-related endocrinopathies is difficult to quantify accurately because of disparities in the diagnosis and monitoring of endocrine toxicities in clinical trials involving immune checkpoint inhibitors (ICPIs). A recently published meta-analysis of 7551 patients from 38 randomized trials reported that the overall incidence of clinically significant endocrinopathies among patients treated with ICPIs is approximately 10%,[1] the most common being hypothyroidism, hyperthyroidism and hypophysitis.[2] The frequency of specific endocrinopathies varies with different ICPIs, as outlined in Table 4.2, and occurs most commonly with combination therapies.

Disconcertingly, immune-related endocrine toxicities may present similarly and often occur insidiously, causing non-specific symptoms such as nausea, headache, fatigue and visual disturbance. As such, a high index of suspicion is required so as not to miss the diagnosis. In addition,

Table 4.2 Ranges of reported endocrine events among different ICPIs (adapted from González-Rodríguez et al.[2]).

Agent	Any endocrinopathy (%)	Hypothyroid (%)	Hyperthyroid (%)	Hypophysitis (%)	Adrenal insufficiency (%)
Ipilimumab	0–29.0	0–9.0	0–2.8	0–17.4	0–1.6
Pembrolizumab	0–19.2	0–11.5	0–7.7	0–1.2	0–4.3
Nivolumab	0–40.0	0–40.0	0–6.5	0–0.9	0–3.3
Combination ipilimumab + nivolumab	16.7–50.0	4–27.0	0–30.0	0–11.7	0–8.0

it is recommended that prior to each ICPI dose, patients receive a thorough clinical review, with periodic screening blood tests to monitor thyroid function, serum cortisol and blood glucose.

What is hypophysitis and what symptoms does it cause?

Hypophysitis refers to inflammation of the pituitary gland. While the incidence of hypophysitis is rare among the general population, it increases significantly with ICPI therapy, occurring in up to 17.4% of patients receiving treatment with ipilimumab (Table 4.2).[3]

Classically, hypophysitis is thought to affect women of childbearing age, causing symptoms of headache and visual disturbance, whereas immune-related hypophysitis appears predominantly to affect men and visual disturbance is rare.

In addition to these clinical features, hypophysitis invariably results in pituitary dysfunction. As such, rather than causing diagnostic, localizing symptoms, hypophysitis often only presents with features of end-organ dysfunction in one, or sometimes multiple, affected hormonal axes downstream of the pituitary, mimicking other endocrinopathies. The diagnosis of hypophysitis is therefore challenging and requires the amalgamation of a number of investigations to differentiate it from alternative causes of hormonal insufficiency.

How is hypophysitis diagnosed?

The diagnosis of hypophysitis is established by the demonstration of low levels of one or more pituitary hormones, namely ACTH, thyroid-stimulating hormone, follicle-stimulating hormone, luteinizing hormone, growth hormone and prolactin, in association with symptoms, identified by a thorough clinical history and examination, and a history of exposure to ICPI therapy.

Additional laboratory investigations are required to differentiate between the various primary and secondary causes for deficiencies of these hormones and support the diagnosis of hypophysitis (Table 4.3). For example, as shown in Table 4.3, while cortisol is low in pituitary insufficiency, it is also low in primary adrenal insufficiency; measuring serum ACTH can differentiate between primary causes, where ACTH is high, and a secondary pituitary pathology, where ACTH is low.

In addition to measuring levels of circulating hormones, other laboratory-based investigations may also be of use in diagnosing hypophysitis. For example, in patients presenting clinically with adrenal insufficiency (as in the case above), isolated hyponatraemia favours a secondary cause of adrenal insufficiency, as in this setting it is likely to be caused by water retention resulting from the loss of vasopressin antagonism by cortisol, which is deficient in pituitary insufficiency. Conversely, hyponatraemia occurring in association with hyperkalaemia is more indicative of a primary

Table 4.3 Changes in circulating hormone levels as a result of different primary and secondary causes of endocrinopathy.

Condition	Primary cause	Secondary cause
Hypothyroidism		
TSH	Increased	Decreased
Free thyroxine	Decreased	Decreased
Hyperthyroidism		
TSH	Decreased	Increased
Free thyroxine	Increased	Increased
Adrenal insufficiency		
Cortisol	Decreased	Decreased
ACTH	Increased	Decreased
Hypogonadism		
Testosterone/oestrogen	Decreased	Decreased
LH/FSH/GnRH	Increased	Decreased

FSH, follicle-stimulating hormone; GnRH, gonadotropin-releasing hormone; LH, luteinizing hormone; TSH, thyroid-stimulating hormone.

adrenal insufficiency owing to a lack of aldosterone secreted by the kidney. Specialist hormone suppression and stimulation tests, such as the Synacthen test, may also be performed to determine whether a hormone deficiency is due to pathology centrally in the pituitary or peripherally at the level of the secretory gland.

Finally, radiological investigations such as brain MRI and whole body CT may be helpful in both supporting the diagnosis of hypophysitis and excluding alternative causes of hormone insufficiency, such as metastatic infiltration of the pituitary and other endocrine glands. While pituitary MRI may strongly substantiate a diagnosis of immune-related hypophysitis by identifying enhancement and swelling of the gland, these changes may resolve within 2 weeks of onset; thus, a normal MRI does not exclude the diagnosis.

What information would you provide to this patient on discharge?

Owing to the lack of a consistent definition among published trials of what constitutes the resolution of an endocrine event, the extent to which endocrine toxicities are reversible remains uncertain.[2] While the symptoms may be improved through replacement of the deficient hormones, affected endocrine glands are unlikely to regain normal secretory function following an acute immune-related event.[4,5] As such, unlike other immune-related toxicities, endocrine toxicities are likely to be permanent and require lifelong hormone replacement, a complication that is particularly significant with regard to life-threatening adrenal insufficiency.[2]

The normal physiological response to stress is to increase cortisol secretion. This is, however, either impossible or insufficient in patients with adrenal insufficiency; therefore, patient education is essential to avoid adrenal crisis. As such, following diagnosis of adrenal insufficiency all patients should be referred to endocrinology for long-term follow-up and formal steroid education including 'sick day' information prior to discharge. Patients should also be discharged with two vials of intravenous 100 mg hydrocortisone in case of emergency and a steroid emergency card.[6]

Sick day rules for patients following a diagnosis of adrenal insufficiency are as follows:

- Double the normal dose of hydrocortisone for a fever >37.5°C or infection/sepsis requiring antibiotics.

- For severe nausea (often with headache), take 20 mg hydrocortisone orally and sip rehydration/electrolyte fluids.

- On vomiting, use emergency 100 mg hydrocortisone injection immediately then seek medical assistance.

- Take 20 mg hydrocortisone orally immediately after major injury to avoid shock.

How would you manage this patient's subsequent anticancer therapy?

There remains ambiguity regarding the discontinuation or continuation of therapy following endocrine toxicity, particularly when ICPI therapy is effective. Current best clinical practice dictates that in the event that a patient being treated with ICPIs presents acutely with an adrenal crisis, further immunotherapy should be withheld until the patient has been fully resuscitated, sepsis has been excluded and oral steroid replacement therapy has been instigated.[7] Subsequent management remains, however, an area of active discussion in the literature. While some have suggested that ICPI therapy should be discontinued in the event of grade 3 or 4 hypophysitis,[8] others have proposed that treatment decisions should be made on an individual basis.[9]

More recently, it has been reported that ipilimumab-induced hypophysitis may positively predict survival in melanoma patients,[10] leading to the suggestion that resumption of ICPI therapy should not be based solely on the presence of endocrine toxicity. Rather, as all cases of hormone insufficiency may be resolved by hormone replacement, the decision to recommence ICPI therapy should centre on the risk to the patient of discontinuing therapy, particularly in patients whose cancer is being controlled by treatment,[11] so as not to deprive them of the best possible care available.

In the present case, following resolution of his symptoms, and in collaboration with the endocrinologists, the patient was restarted on pembrolizumab, as he was established on oral steroid maintenance and was responding to treatment. He continued to tolerate treatment with no further toxicity and ultimately achieved a complete response.

Conclusion and learning points

- Be vigilant:
  - Endocrine toxicities such as adrenal insufficiency may be life-threatening. Furthermore, immune-related endocrine toxicities may all present similarly and insidiously; therefore, a high index of suspicion and a low threshold for investigation/treatment are required so as not to miss them.
- Perform screening investigations:
  - Patients should undergo a thorough clinical review prior to each ICPI dose, as well as screening blood tests to monitor thyroid function, serum cortisol and blood glucose periodically during treatment.

- Hormone deficiencies are often permanent:
  - Patients often require lifelong hormone replacement therapy; therefore, collaboration with endocrinologists is essential for patient quality of life and wellbeing.
- Treatment cessation is not mandatory:
  - Once an acute event has resolved and the patient is established on hormone replacement therapy, ICPI therapy may be recommended following consideration of the risks of continuing therapy against the risks of discontinuing therapy at an individual patient level, in collaboration with both the patient and the endocrinologist.

References

1   Barroso-Sousa R, Barry WT, Garrido-Castro AC, *et al.* Incidence of endocrine dysfunction following the use of different immune checkpoint inhibitor regimens: a systematic review and meta-analysis. *JAMA Oncol* 2018; 4: 173–82.

2   González-Rodríguez E, Rodríguez-Abreu D, Spanish Group for Cancer Immuno-Biotherapy (GETICA). Immune checkpoint inhibitors: review and management of endocrine adverse events. *Oncologist* 2016; 21: 804–16.

3   Maker AV, Yang JC, Sherry RM, *et al.* Intrapatient dose escalation of anti-CTLA-4 antibody in patients with metastatic melanoma. *J Immunother* 2006; 29: 455–63.

4   Larkin J, Chiarion-Sileni V, González R, *et al.* Combined nivolumab and ipilimumab or monotherapy in untreated melanoma. *N Engl J Med* 2015; 373: 23–34.

5   Sznol M, Postow MA, Davies MJ, *et al.* Endocrine-related adverse events associated with immune checkpoint blockade and expert insights on their management. *Cancer Treat Rev* 2017; 58: 70–6.

6   Arlt W, Society for Endocrinology Clinical Committee. Society for Endocrinology endocrine emergency guidance: emergency management of acute adrenal insufficiency (adrenal crisis) in adult patients. *Endocr Connect* 2016; 5: G1–3.

7   Brahmer JR, Lacchetti C, Schneider BJ, *et al.* Management of immune-related adverse events in patients treated with immune checkpoint inhibitor therapy: American Society of Clinical Oncology clinical practice guideline. *J Clin Oncol* 2018; 36: 1714–68.

8   Torino F, Corsello SM, Salvatori R. Endocrinological side-effects of immune checkpoint inhibitors. *Curr Opin Oncol* 2016; 28: 278–87.

9   Corsello SM, Barnabei A, Marchetti P, *et al.* Endocrine side effects induced by immune checkpoint inhibitors. *J Clin Endocrinol Metab* 2013; 98: 1361–75.

10 Faje AT, Sullivan R, Lawrence D, *et al.* Ipilimumab-induced hypophysitis: a detailed longitudinal analysis in a large cohort of patients with metastatic melanoma. *J Clin Endocrinol Metab* 2014; 99: 4078–85.

11 Illouz F, Briet C, Cloix L, *et al.* Endocrine toxicity of immune checkpoint inhibitors: essential crosstalk between endocrinologists and oncologists. *Cancer Med* 2017; 6: 1923–9.

05 Immune Checkpoint Inhibitors in Patients with Autoimmune Disease

Alfred C.P. So, Ruth E. Board

Case history

 A 65-year-old woman with a history of seronegative arthritis presented to her rheumatology follow-up with night sweats, lethargy, lower back pain and discomfort when lying down. Her medical history included cutaneous melanoma, hypertension and hypercholesterolaemia. A superficial, spreading non-ulcerated 1.2 mm (pT2a) malignant melanoma had been excised from her left thigh 28 years earlier. Her arthritis was well controlled with hydroxychloroquine only. A CT scan revealed metastatic lesions in the retroperitoneum, left external iliac nodes and pelvic sidewalls. Biopsies confirmed recurrence of a *BRAF* V600E mutant melanoma. Her performance status was 0. Detailed discussions took place with the patient about the risks and benefits of starting immunotherapy vs serine/threonine-protein kinase B-Raf (BRAF)-targeted therapy. The patient decided to proceed with primary treatment with pembrolizumab 200 mg/kg every 3 weeks.

After cycle 1 she experienced grade 2 arthritis and required treatment with prednisolone 30 mg once daily tapered over 4 weeks. A partial response to treatment was confirmed by CT scan 12 weeks after starting treatment. She continued to experience grades 1–2 exacerbations of her arthritis throughout her treatment course, requiring intermittent steroid dosing. Ultimately, she was kept on a maintenance dose of prednisolone 10 mg once daily, which controlled her arthritis symptoms. She was later diagnosed with osteoporosis plus sacral stress fractures and was started on bisphosphonates. She has currently completed 31 cycles of pembrolizumab, with no treatment deferrals. Follow-up CT scans continue to demonstrate response to immunotherapy.

What is the evidence for the safety of immune checkpoint inhibitors (ICPIs) in patients with pre-existing autoimmune disease?

Do patients with pre-existing autoimmune disease have a poorer clinical outcome with anti-programmed cell death protein 1 (PD-1) therapy?

What are the treatment options for our patient's flare of arthritis?

Can we predict which patients are likely to have severe exacerbations of their autoimmune disease?

How should at-risk patients be managed by the multidisciplinary team?

What is the evidence for the safety of ICPIs in patients with pre-existing autoimmune disease?

Clinical trials of immunotherapy have excluded patients with pre-existing autoimmune disease, owing to the potential risk of severe exacerbations related to immune activation. Currently, there are only a small number of retrospective studies detailing the use of immunotherapy in these settings.[1-3]

Johnson *et al.*[1] carried out an international multicentre retrospective study of 30 patients with advanced melanoma and pre-existing autoimmune disease receiving ipilimumab. The median age of the patients was 59.5 years (range 30–80 years) and 26 (87%) had stage IV M1c disease. Prior to ipilimumab treatment, 13 patients (43%) were receiving active systemic treatment for their autoimmune disease. Eight patients (27%) had grades 3–5 exacerbations requiring systemic steroids and 10 patients (33%) experienced a new immune-related adverse event (irAE). The duration to autoimmune disease exacerbation was most common between weeks 2 and 3 and at week 6 (range 3 days to 7 months). One patient died from autoimmune colitis unrelated to his pre-existing autoimmune disease.

Menzies *et al.*[2] carried out an international multicentre retrospective study of 52 patients with advanced melanoma and pre-existing autoimmune disease receiving anti-PD-1 inhibitors. The median age of the patients was 71 years (range 23–88 years) and 44 (85%) had stage IV M1c disease. Prior to anti-PD-1 therapy, 20 patients (38%) were receiving immunosuppressive treatment for their autoimmune disease. Twenty-eight patients (54%) had previously been treated with ipilimumab; the majority of patients received pembrolizumab. Twenty patients (38%) had an autoimmune exacerbation requiring systemic treatment, three of whom had a grade 3 exacerbation. Two patients (4%) permanently discontinued anti-PD-1 therapy because of their autoimmune exacerbation. Fifteen patients (29%) developed new irAEs. Median duration to autoimmune flare-up was 38 days (range 8–161 days).

In Germany, Gutzmer *et al.*[3] carried out a multicentre retrospective study of 19 patients with advanced melanoma and pre-existing autoimmune disease receiving anti-PD-1 therapy. The median age of the patients was 54 years (range 38–76 years). Twelve patients (63%) were receiving systemic treatment for their autoimmune disease, six of whom were on hormone replacement therapy (i.e. levothyroxine, hydrocortisone). Eight patients (42%) had an autoimmune exacerbation requiring treatment, two of whom experienced a grade 3 exacerbation. Three patients (16%) had new irAEs. Autoimmune flare-ups occurred between weeks 3 and 20 after starting anti-PD-1 therapy.

Although these studies suggest that ICPIs may be safely administered to patients with pre-existing autoimmune disease, their small sample sizes mean that the results should still be interpreted with caution. The study populations were heterogeneous, having varying autoimmune diseases ranging from rheumatological to neurological conditions. Interestingly, autoimmune exacerbations may be more common in patients with rheumatological conditions. Of the patients with pre-existing rheumatological conditions, flare-ups occurred in six out of 14 (43%), 14 out of 27 (52%) and five out of nine patients (56%), respectively.[1-3]

Do patients with pre-existing autoimmune disease have a poorer clinical outcome with anti-PD-1 therapy?

The overall response rate to anti-PD-1 therapy in the retrospective studies described above (32–33%) was comparable to that achieved in the pivotal trials KEYNOTE-002 (21.1%),[4] KEYNOTE-006 (32.9%)[5] and CheckMate 067 (43.7%).[6] In the study of Menzies *et al.*,[2] median progression-free survival (PFS) was 6.2 months (95% CI 4.2, 8.2). The majority of the patients received pembrolizumab. This was similar to the median PFS of 5.4 months (95% CI 4.7, 6.0) and 4.1 months (95% CI 2.9, 6.9), respectively, in the KEYNOTE-002 and KEYNOTE-006 trials.[4,5] Based on the limited evidence available, patients with pre-existing autoimmune diseases do not appear to have poorer survival outcomes compared with those without autoimmunity. Autoimmune exacerbations do not seem to correlate with overall response rate in those retrospective studies.[2,3] On the contrary, a recent multicentre retrospective study in France of 112 patients with pre-existing autoimmune diseases suggested that PFS was longer in those who experienced flares of their disease or other unrelated irAEs. This gain in survival appeared to be lost when these patients were treated with immunosuppressive agents.[7]

Generally, irAEs may be safely managed without reversing the treatment's anti-tumour response but may depend on the immunosuppressive agent used.[1-3] Caution is advised in using less conventional immunomodulatory drugs that target specific pathways. A case study observed loss of anti-tumour response from interleukin (IL)-17 blockade to reverse the exacerbation of a patient's psoriasis and Crohn's disease after anti-PD-1 therapy.[8] Interestingly, another case study demonstrated that concurrent treatment with pembrolizumab and tocilizumab (an IL-6 inhibitor) safely limited the exacerbation of Crohn's disease without loss of anti-tumour response.[9]

What are the treatment options for our patient's flare of arthritis?

Our patient experienced grades 1–2 exacerbations of her inflammatory arthritis throughout her treatment course. The evidence surrounding the management of immune-related arthralgia is primarily based on expert opinion and small observational studies, and is even more limited in patients with pre-existing arthritis. These studies[1-3] have demonstrated, however, that patients with pre-existing autoimmune disease may be adequately managed with steroids and steroid-sparing agents. The European Society for Medical Oncology (ESMO) guidelines for the management of toxicities of immunotherapy recommend stepwise management of immune-related arthralgia, starting with paracetamol and NSAIDs for grade 1 arthralgia.[10] Low-dose steroids (e.g. prednisolone 10–20 mg once daily) or intra-articular steroid injections may be used for grade 2 arthralgia refractory to simple analgesics. Higher doses (i.e. prednisolone 0.5–1.0 mg/kg once daily) are recommended for grade 3 arthralgia; ICPIs should be stopped at this point. Re-introduction of ICPIs may be considered later.

Can we predict which patients are likely to have severe exacerbations of their autoimmune disease?

Currently, there are no validated prognostic factors or biomarkers to determine which patients will have severe exacerbations of their autoimmune disease. Menzies et al.[2] observed that patients with active symptoms prior to anti-PD-1 therapy had more frequent exacerbations compared with those with inactive disease (60% vs 30%, respectively; $p=0.039$). It should be noted that there was selection bias in these studies,[1-3] since patients with more severe autoimmune diseases might not have been offered ICPIs, owing to limited safety information about their conditions. More caution may be needed in patients requiring significant immunosuppressive agents in whom a flare of the condition may be more difficult to control. Although the baseline activity of autoimmune diseases may be a potential predictor of future exacerbations, autoimmunity tends to have a relapsing–remitting course. Appreciating a patient's full history of the autoimmune disease may help better predict the response to ICPI treatment. Treatment response may be guided by trends in validated disease severity scores, such as the DAS28 for rheumatoid arthritis, and early involvement of the rheumatologist. Potential future biomarkers for predicting toxicity to ICPIs may include serum eosinophils and IL-17.[11] A full discussion of the risks and benefits of immunotherapy vs the risk of autoimmune disease flare should be had; for example, there may be a more significant and potentially permanent and catastrophic impact with flare of neurological autoimmune conditions such as Guillain–Barré syndrome compared with flare of mild rheumatoid arthritis.

How should at-risk patients be managed by the multidisciplinary team?

First of all, a patient's full medical background should be elicited from first point of contact. This includes when the autoimmune disease was diagnosed, current and previous treatments, and current control of the condition. A thorough discussion should be held with the patient regarding the risk of autoimmune flare-ups with ICPIs; prior to starting immunotherapy, the patient should be educated about how to manage side effects and whom to contact if irAEs occur. In the case of severe exacerbations requiring hospital assessment, the acute oncology team should be contacted as soon as possible and treatment initiated following any local guidance and validated national/international standards (e.g. ESMO guidance). Consideration should be given to prescribing a short course of oral steroids (e.g. prednisolone 30 mg once daily) for patients to take home after immunotherapy treatment for some conditions. Patients should be encouraged to contact the hospital prior to starting any steroids. Our patient was given an anticipatory prescription of prednisone 30 mg once daily, which proved to be very useful in reducing pain from her flare of arthritis in order to facilitate travel to an outpatient review. Her flare management was coordinated via a 24 h telephone helpline.

Patients at risk of autoimmune flares should have frequent review, especially at the start of their treatment course. Review could be achieved through a combination of telephone (with a specialist nurse) and clinic follow-ups. There should be early involvement of the primary physician overseeing the patient's autoimmune disease (i.e. rheumatologist, dermatologist, neurologist), to gain further insight into the severity of the disease and seek advice regarding the management of future flare-ups.

Finally, to allow full coordination of care, the patient's primary care physician should be made aware of the treatment the patient is receiving, the potential side effects and the different specialties involved in the patient's care.

Conclusion and learning points

- ICPIs appear to be safe to use in patients with pre-existing autoimmune disease.
- Having an autoimmune disease and flare-ups from ICPI treatment does not reduce survival outcomes.
- Autoimmune flare-ups may be safely managed with steroids and steroid-sparing agents.
- Consider prescribing steroids prior to treatment initiation in case of future flare-ups.
- Patient education is vital to optimize the management of autoimmune flare-ups.
- Early involvement of the physician overseeing the patient's autoimmune disease is advised.

References

1 Johnson DB, Sullivan RJ, Ott PA, *et al*. Ipilimumab therapy in patients with advanced melanoma and preexisting autoimmune disorders. *JAMA Oncol* 2016; 2: 234–40.

2 Menzies AM, Johnson DB, Ramanujam S, *et al*. Anti-PD-1 therapy in patients with advanced melanoma and preexisting autoimmune disorders or major toxicity with ipilimumab. *Ann Oncol* 2017; 28: 368–76.

3 Gutzmer R, Koop A, Meier F, *et al*. Programmed cell death protein-1 (PD-1) inhibitor therapy in patients with advanced melanoma and preexisting autoimmunity or ipilimumab-triggered autoimmunity. *Eur J Cancer* 2017; 75: 24–32.

4 Ribas A, Puzanov I, Dummer R, *et al*. Pembrolizumab versus investigator-choice chemotherapy for ipilimumab-refractory melanoma (KEYNOTE-002): a randomised, controlled, phase 2 trial. *Lancet Oncol* 2015; 16: 908–18.

5 Robert C, Schachter J, Long GV, *et al*. Pembrolizumab versus ipilimumab in advanced melanoma. *N Engl J Med* 2015; 372: 2521–32.

6 Larkin J, Chiarion-Sileni V, Gonzalez R, *et al*. Combined nivolumab and ipilimumab or monotherapy in untreated melanoma. *N Engl J Med* 2015; 373: 23–34.

7 Tison A, Quere G, Misery L, *et al*. OP0196 Safety and efficacy of immune checkpoint inhibitors in patients with cancer and preexisting autoimmune diseases: a nationwide multicenter retrospective study. *Ann Rheum Dis* 2018; 77: 147.

8 Esfahani K, Miller Jr WH. Reversal of autoimmune toxicity and loss of tumour response by interleukin-17 blockade. *N Engl J Med* 2017; 376: 1989–91.

9 Uemura M, Trinh VA, Haymaker C, *et al*. Selective inhibition of autoimmune exacerbation while preserving the anti-tumor clinical benefit using IL-6 blockade in a patient with advanced melanoma and Crohn's disease: a case report. *J Hematol Oncol* 2016; 9: 81.

10 Haanen JBAG, Carbonnel F, Robert C, *et al*. Management of toxicities from immunotherapy: ESMO clinical practice guidelines for diagnosis, treatment and follow-up. *Ann Oncol* 2017; 28 (suppl 4): iv119–42.

11 Hopkins AM, Rowland A, Kichenadasse G, *et al*. Predicting response and toxicity to immune checkpoint inhibitors using routinely available blood and clinical markers. *Br J Cancer* 2017; 117: 913–20.

Further reading

- Abdel-Wahab N, Shah M, Lopez-Olivo MA, Suarez-Almazor ME. Use of immune checkpoint inhibitors in the treatment of patients with cancer and preexisting autoimmune disease. *Ann Intern Med* 2018; 168: 121–30.

- UK Oncology Nursing Society (2018). *Acute oncology initial management guidelines. Version 2.0*. Available from: https://az659834.vo.msecnd.net/eventsairwesteuprod/production-succinct-public/e80a54a0570a470bb0cf1ab07a7644e7 (accessed 17 July 2018).

CASE STUDY

06 A Patient with Lung Cancer Who Received an Immune Checkpoint Inhibitor in the First Line Setting

Adam P. Januszewski, Sanjay Popat

Case history

A 69-year-old woman with an 8 week history of persistent cough and chest pain associated with a 2 kg weight loss was referred for urgent assessment. Investigations identified a 66 mm right upper lobe lung mass adjacent to the pleura with mediastinal and mesenteric lymphadenopathy and a sclerotic lesion at T3 vertebral body. Percutaneous CT-guided biopsy of the thoracic mass demonstrated a poorly differentiated *TTF1*-positive adenocarcinoma with features of sarcomatoid dedifferentiation. Her medical history included a hiatus hernia and type 2 diabetes mellitus. Her father had been diagnosed with lung cancer at the age of 66. She was a cleaner, married with two children and a smoker with an 80 pack-year history.

The thoracic multidisciplinary team recommended systemic therapy with palliative intent for pT3cN3cM1c non-small-cell lung carcinoma (NSCLC) adenocarcinoma subtype and she was referred to medical oncology. Further molecular testing demonstrated *EGFR* and *ALK* wild-type; 100% of tumour cells stained positive for programmed death-ligand 1 (PD-L1) by immunohistochemistry using the 22C3 clone (Dako Agilent, Santa Clara, CA, USA), rendering her suitable for consideration for first line pembrolizumab immune checkpoint inhibitor (ICPI) therapy.

She commenced pembrolizumab monotherapy and after three cycles of treatment her CT response assessment evaluation scan demonstrated a partial response (right upper lobe mass reduced by 60% and regression of lymphadenopathy). She continued on pembrolizumab but developed increasing dyspnoea after the fifth cycle. A CT scan identified pneumonitis (grade 2), for which she was commenced on prednisolone. Her pembrolizumab was paused and restarted after completing a steroid wean. She continues to receive pembrolizumab with an ongoing partial response 7 months after commencing treatment.

What is the evidence base for using ICPI therapy in the first line setting for patients with NSCLC?

What are the clinical characteristics of patients who respond to ICPIs?

What are the contraindications to ICPIs and for which treatment-related toxicities should the patient with lung cancer give consent?

How may the efficacy of ICPIs for patients with lung cancer be enhanced?

What is the evidence base for using ICPI therapy in the first line setting for patients with NSCLC?

Platinum-based doublet systemic chemotherapy is the standard of care for metastatic NSCLC.[1] In recent years the identification of oncogenic drivers (*EGFR, ALK, ROS*) in patients with lung cancer has meant the development of new targeted agents, which has improved outcomes. In the majority of patients with non-oncogene-addicted NSCLC, however, there have been no major advances in systemic treatment until the advent of ICPI therapy.

The benefit of the ICPIs nivolumab and pembrolizumab in lung cancer was initially demonstrated in the relapsed (second line and beyond) setting and subsequently (as in this case) for use in the first line setting (Table 6.1)

KEYNOTE-024

In KEYNOTE-024 (ClinicalTrials.gov NCT02142738), 305 patients with metastatic NSCLC (with no *EGFR* or *ALK* somatic aberrations) expressing PD-L1 by immunohistochemistry in >50% of cells were randomly stratified to receive pembrolizumab or investigator-choice platinum-based doublet chemotherapy.[2] Those who received pembrolizumab had a larger overall response rate (44.8% vs 27.8%; p=0.0011), longer median progression-free survival (PFS) (10.3 vs 6 months; HR 0.50; 95% CI 0.37, 0.68; $p<0.001$) and longer median overall survival (OS) (30 vs 14.2 months; HR 0.63; 95% CI 0.47, 0.86; p=0.002). Since publication of these findings, pembrolizumab has become standard of care for such patients.

CheckMate 026

CheckMate 026 (ClinicalTrials.gov NCT02041533) is a phase III trial contemporaneous to KEYNOTE-024, which tested the efficacy of nivolumab in 541 patients with metastatic NSCLC and no *EGFR* or *ALK* somatic aberrations.[3] Patients with PD-L1 levels >1% were randomized to receive nivolumab or investigator-choice platinum-based chemotherapy. Nivolumab did not demonstrate

Table 6.1 Trials of ICPIs of patients with NSCLC in the first line setting.

Variable	KEYNOTE-024[2]	CheckMate 026[3]
Investigational drug	Pembrolizumab	Nivolumab
Comparator regimen	Carboplatin/pemetrexed (44%)	Carboplatin/pemetrexed (44%)
	Cisplatin/pemetrexed (24%)	Cisplatin/pemetrexed (33%)
	Carboplatin/gemcitabine (13%)	Carboplatin/gemcitabine (13%)
	Carboplatin/paclitaxel (11%)	Cisplatin/gemcitabine (5%)
	Cisplatin/gemcitabine (7%)	Carboplatin/paclitaxel (6%)
Median OS	Not reached at time of publication	14.4 months (vs 13.2)
	OS at 6 months 80.2% vs 72.4%	HR 1.02 (p=NS)
	HR 0.60 (p=0.005)	
Median PFS	10.3 months (vs 6)	4.2 months (vs 5.9)
	HR 0.50 ($p<0.001$)	HR 1.15 (p=0.25)
Overall response rate	44.8% (vs 27.8%)	26% (vs 33%)

improved PFS (median PFS 4.2 vs 5.9 months; HR 1.15; 95% CI 0.91, 1.45) or OS (in patients with PD-L1 >5% median OS 14.4 vs 13.2 months; HR 1.02; 95% CI 0.80, 1.30). As a consequence, nivolumab monotherapy has not been taken forward for use in the first line setting, although it has been further developed in combination trials.

Optimal first line treatment of patients with NSCLC of any histology with a PD-L1 expression >50% (except those with *EGFR* or *ALK* alterations, for whom molecular target therapy remains the standard) is currently pembrolizumab monotherapy. Despite proposed similar mechanisms of action it is unclear why the outcomes of these two trials were different, but the reason is likely related to patient selection, biomarker stratification and trial design, rather than innate differences between drugs. For patients with PD-L1 expression <50%, however, the standard of care remains systemic platinum-based doublet chemotherapy, although trials are ongoing investigating methods to improve the efficacy of ICPIs, both in those with and those without PD-L1 expression, usually by combining agents with chemotherapy.

What are the clinical characteristics of patients who respond to ICPIs?

Patients with PD-L1 expression >50% are more likely to respond to first line pembrolizumab than to platinum-based doublet chemotherapy and therefore derive a survival benefit. Although in the relapsed (second line) setting, expression of PD-L1 >1% is the licensed indication for pembrolizumab, both nivolumab and atezolizumab have demonstrated a survival advantage over docetaxel monotherapy in patients without PD-L1 expression. Hence, PD-L1 expression testing is not mandatory to prescribe these therapies. Given that the magnitude of survival benefit seems to be related to the level of PD-L1 expression, however, it may still be a clinically useful parameter. Interpreting the clinical outcomes of trials in patients receiving ICPI therapy is also complicated by variation in antibody-staining sensitivity observed across anti-PD-L1 monoclonal clones. Newer predictive biomarkers such as tumour mutational burden[4] may potentially be used to better predict response to ICPIs in the future but is not yet an approved biomarker to implement in routine clinical decision making.

High expression of PD-L1 (>50%) was observed in 30% of NSCLC patients screened in KEY-NOTE-024. A meta-analysis of 11,444 patients showed that PD-L1 expression was associated with a poorer prognosis (HR 1.40; 95% CI 1.19, 1.65; $p<0.001$).[5] In a pooled analysis, PD-L1 status was associated with sex, smoking status, histology, differentiation, tumour size, lymph node metastasis, TNM stage and *EGFR* mutation (Table 6.2).[5] In the present case the patient had a significant

Table 6.2 Clinicopathological associations with PD-L1 expression.[5]		
Clinicopathological feature	Odds ratio (95% CI)	*p*-value
Male	1.46 (1.24, 1.71)	<0.001
Smoker	1.57 (1.28, 1.93)	<0.001
Squamous histology	1.59 (1.11, 2.26)	0.01
High histological grade	2.55 (2.05, 3.19)	<0.001
Larger tumour size	1.70 (1.29, 2.25)	<0.001
Lymph node metastasis	1.34 (1.19, 1.50)	<0.001
TNM staging	1.45 (1.18, 1.78)	<0.001

smoking history and a large high-grade tumour in the context of advanced disease, both raising the likelihood of higher PD-L1 level.

What are the contraindications to ICPIs and for which treatment–related toxicities should the patient with lung cancer give consent?

Toxicities of ICPIs may develop in any organ system because of effector T cell activity against autoantigens, although they are most frequent in skin, colon, endocrine organs, liver and lung. These immune-related adverse events (irAEs) vary in incidence and severity depending on the class of ICPI, i.e. cytotoxic T lymphocyte-associated protein 4 (CTLA-4) or programmed cell death protein 1 (PD-1)/PD-L1 targeting. While not an absolute contraindication, significant care should be taken when considering treatment of patients with autoimmune conditions, owing to the risk of life-threatening/fatal flare. As patients receiving disease-modifying therapy for an autoimmune condition taking 10 mg prednisolone equivalent at baseline or with organ transplantation were excluded from registration trials of ICPIs, the risk:benefit ratio has not been prospectively evaluated.

Compared with platinum-based doublet chemotherapy, pembrolizumab was associated with fewer total adverse events of any grade (73.4% vs 90.0%) and fewer higher-grade adverse events in the first line setting (grade ≥ 3, 26.6% vs 53.3%). For irAEs, 9.7% of patients experienced grades 3–5 events, including skin reactions (3.9%) and pneumonitis (2.6%). While the incidence of pneumonitis is similar between cases of NSCLC and melanoma, the rate of treatment-related deaths is higher in NSCLC.

ICPIs appear to have fewer toxicities compared with platinum-based doublet chemotherapy, although irAEs may be long term, unlike chemotherapy-related adverse events, which are mostly haematological and self limiting. Therefore, it is important to account for irAEs when consenting patients to ICPI treatment. While ICPI combinations may improve outcomes, the breadth of toxicities and their additive effects need consideration, as they may also increase clinically meaningful treatment-related toxicities in both frequency and severity.

How may the efficacy of ICPIs for patients with lung cancer be enhanced?

Immunotherapy monotherapy is only beneficial to a select group of patients. Therefore, trials investigating the effect of combining ICPIs with other ICPIs, chemotherapy, targeted agents and other modalities such as radiotherapy are currently enrolling. The principle of combining treatments is to either combine agents with synergistic effect or to enhance the immunogenicity of 'cold' tumours. A number of these studies will report in 2018–2019.

KEYNOTE-189 (ClinicalTrials.gov NCT02578680) and CheckMate 227 (ClinicalTrials.gov NCT02477826) are the first phase III studies of ICPI combination, and ICPI and chemotherapy combination, in the first line setting. KEYNOTE-189 is evaluating the impact of adding pembrolizumab to first line chemotherapy for patients with non-squamous NSCLC. Median OS has not been reached in the ICPI combination arm at the time of publication, although the HR for death is 0.49 (95% CI 0.38, 0.64; $p<0.001$) when the ICPI chemotherapy combination is compared with the placebo chemotherapy combination. Benefit is demonstrated regardless of PD-L1 status. CheckMate 227 is evaluating several therapy combinations including the efficacy of combination ICPIs in the first line NSCLC setting. Early reports of the results of these studies may have the potential to change the standard of care of patients with lung cancer in the first line setting.

Conclusion and learning points

- The ICPI pembrolizumab has demonstrated improved OS when compared with platinum-based doublet chemotherapy regimens and is now the standard of care for patients with NSCLC (any histology except *EGFR*- and *ALK*-oncogene addicted) who express high levels of PD-L1 (>50%).

- PD-L1 is our best biomarker to predict response to ICPIs; the likelihood of having high expression is associated with sex, smoking status, histology, differentiation, tumour size, lymph node metastasis and TNM stage.

- While pneumonitis and skin reactions are the most common severe irAEs (grade ≥3), trial data suggest that pembrolizumab has reduced toxicities compared with chemotherapy. This should, however, be taken in the context of the different nature and duration of these side effects, which may be long term.

- Numerous trials are underway investigating combinations of ICPIs and with chemotherapy or radiotherapy, with the aim to improve their efficacy. The results of these are awaited and may lead to further changes in the treatment of lung cancer in the first line setting.

References

1 Non-small Cell Lung Cancer Collaborative Group. Chemotherapy in non-small cell lung cancer: a meta-analysis using updated data on individual patients from 52 randomised clinical trials. *BMJ* 1995; 311: 899–909.

2 Reck M, Rodríguez-Abreu D, Robinson AG, *et al.* Pembrolizumab versus chemotherapy for PD-L1-positive non-small-cell lung cancer. *N Engl J Med* 2016; 375: 1823–33.

3 Carbone DP, Reck M, Paz-Ares L, *et al.* First-line nivolumab in stage IV or recurrent non-small-cell lung cancer. *N Engl J Med* 2017; 376: 2415–26.

4 Goodman AM, Kato S, Bazhenova L, *et al.* Tumor mutational burden as an independent predictor of response to immunotherapy in diverse cancers. *Mol Cancer Ther* 2017; 16: 2598–608.

5 Zhang M, Li G, Wang Y, *et al.* PD-L1 expression in lung cancer and its correlation with driver mutations: a meta-analysis. *Sci Rep* 2017; 7: 10255.

Further reading

- Aguiar PN Jr, De Mello RA, Barreto CMN, *et al.* Immune checkpoint inhibitors for advanced non-small cell lung cancer: emerging sequencing for new treatment targets. *ESMO Open* 2017; 2: e000200.

- Assi HI, Kamphorst AO, Moukalled NM, Ramalingam SS. Immune checkpoint inhibitors in advanced non-small cell lung cancer. *Cancer* 2018; 124: 248–61.

- Wu J, Hong D, Zhang X, *et al.* PD-1 inhibitors increase the incidence and risk of pneumonitis in cancer patients in a dose-independent manner: a meta-analysis. *Sci Rep* 2017; 7: 44173.

07 Sinonasal Mucosal Malignant Melanoma

Anna Olsson-Brown, Joseph Sacco

Case history

A 72-year-old Caucasian woman with locally advanced sinonasal mucosal malignant melanoma (MMM) received combination immunotherapy. She had initially presented with apparent nasal polyps, which were resected but which were shown to be melanoma on pathological review. Imaging showed extensive malignancy involving the left nasal cavity and ethmoid sinus with extension into the maxillary sinus. Multidisciplinary team discussion confirmed her malignancy was inoperable and she was referred to the medical oncology team for consideration of systemic therapy.

Mutational analysis showed no evidence of a *BRAF* V600 mutation in the tumour and she was commenced on combination cytotoxic T lymphocyte-associated protein 4 (CTLA-4) and programmed cell death protein 1 (PD-1) immune checkpoint inhibitor (ICPI) therapy with ipilimumab and nivolumab.

After three cycles of combination therapy she experienced mild fatigue and was found to have isolated adrenal impairment with hypocortisolaemia. Her pituitary axes remained intact. Given her minimal symptoms, she received hydrocortisone replacement and continued with immunotherapy. An initial CT scan after four cycles of combination immunotherapy showed a significant reduction in the size of the left nasal tumour to practical resolution. Given her stability on hormone replacement and response to therapy, she progressed to maintenance single-agent nivolumab.

Following one cycle of single-agent therapy (five ICPI cycles in total) the patient became acutely unwell with nausea, dizziness and confusion. On admission to hospital she was found to have unrecordably high blood glucose with significant acidosis and a high lactate. She was diagnosed with diabetic ketoacidosis and managed according to acute protocols. She was admitted to the ITU and improved within 24 h. She was discharged from hospital after a 5 day stay having been started on long-term basal–bolus insulin therapy. Given how unwell she had been with multiple immune-related adverse events (irAEs), she did not receive any further ICPI treatment and commenced active surveillance.

Follow-up imaging a year after commencing ICPIs showed a complete response to treatment. A subsequent scan 10 months after discontinuation of therapy, however, suggested mild thickening on the left sinonasal cavity, confirmed as recurrence on an interval MRI scan. The patient underwent surgical resection of the recurrent melanoma with planned consolidation radiotherapy.

This patient experienced an initial response to combination immunotherapy, with a period of complete response amounting to 15 months of disease control. Furthermore, she underwent surgical resection following ICPI therapy despite initially having inoperable disease.

What is the clinical landscape in MMM?

What is the role of ICPIs in MMM?

What endocrinopathies can be caused by ICPIs?

What is the recommended management of diabetes secondary to ICPI therapy?

What is the clinical landscape in MMM?

MMM arises in the epithelial lining of multiple organs. It is rare, accounting for ~1% of the total melanoma population. In contrast to cutaneous melanoma (CM), the incidence of MMM over the last decade has been stable.[1] There is a female predominance and the median age of onset is 70 years (although MMM arising in the oral cavity tends to present at a younger age).[2,3] There are, however, no clear predisposing factors. MMM commonly arises in the nasal cavity, paranasal sinuses, oral cavity, rectum, anus, vulva and vagina.[1] Other less common sites include the larynx, pharynx, urinary tract and small intestine. More than 20% of cases are associated with multiple foci of disease and 40% are amelanocytic.[4]

MMM is an aggressive subset of melanoma that is associated with a worse prognosis compared with its cutaneous counterparts.[4] Five year overall survival (OS) for CM is 80% compared with 25% in MMM.[1] This difference is likely to be multifactorial but it is known that MMM is broadly associated with late presentation. It is also difficult to stage-match MMM and CM given that there are different staging systems, and apparently similar stages may not reflect a similar stage of disease.

The disparate origins of MMM have led to the production of numerous staging systems. The most widely recognized system is that of the American Joint Committee on Cancer (AJCC), which was developed for use in MMM of the head and neck but is often applied to lesions arising from other sites.[5] MMM of the head and neck is classified as stage III or stage IV and is then categorized depending on whether it is clinically localized or displays regional nodal involvement or distant metastatic disease. The AJCC categorization is shown in Table 7.1.[5]

Head and neck MMM

There is a differential distribution in the different anatomical sites of the head and neck. The most common sites of origin are the oral cavity (22%) and the nasal cavity, turbinates and sinuses (69%); the pharynx, larynx and upper oesophagus are less frequently involved (9%).[6] Local disease is assessed via endoscopic examination and CT or MRI imaging of the primary disease. CT or PET-CT is generally carried out to detect distant metastases. Regional lymph nodes are identified in 15% of patients with MMM of the oral cavity and 6% of patients with sinonasal disease.[1]

The mainstay of treatment is complete excision in stage III/IVA disease, often followed by adjuvant radiotherapy. Lymph node dissection is not recommended in sinonasal disease, given that less than 10% of cases are associated with nodal spread. Conversely, 25% of MMMs of the oral cavity have lymph node involvement; therefore, lymph node dissection is a standard element of surgical resection in this group.[7] Local recurrence is very common even in the case of complete

Table 7.1 AJCC staging of MMM of the head and neck.[5]

Clinical extent of disease prior to treatment	Stage category definition
Primary tumour	
T3	Mucosal disease only
T4a	Moderately advanced disease involving deep soft tissues, cartilage, bone or overlying skin
T4b	Very advanced disease Tumour involving brain, dura, skull base, lower cranial nerves, masticator space, carotid arteries, prevertebral space or mediastinal structures
Regional lymph nodes	
NX	Cannot be assessed
N0	No regional lymph node metastasis
N1	Regional lymph node metastasis present
Distant metastasis	
M0	No distant metastasis
M1	Distant metastasis
Clinical stage	
Stage III	T3N0M0
Stage IVA	T4aN0M0/T3aN1M0/T4aN1M0
Stage IVB	T4bAnyNM0
Stage IVC	AnyT/AnyN/M1

surgical resection; risk factors for recurrence include incomplete resection, tumour size and the presence of vascular invasion.[7,8] The median time to recurrence is 6–12 months from surgical intervention.[8]

If surgery is not feasible then radical radiotherapy is often considered and is associated with tumour control rates of 61–85%; however, the vast majority of tumours progress after a period of stability.[7] The optimal dosing and fractionation of radiotherapy are yet to be established. Local disease recurrence is very commonly associated with distant metastasis; disease recurrence is treated in line with treatment for locally advanced or metastatic CM.

Vulvovaginal and anorectal MMM

MMM accounts for 9% of vulval malignancies and 3% of vaginal malignancies.[9] While there are no established risk factors, chronic inflammatory diseases, chemical irritants, viral pathogens and genetic factors are all thought to potentially be involved.[10] Surgical wide local excision (the extent of which is driven by primary tumour size) is the mainstay of treatment, but, as with head and neck lesions, recurrence and/or metastasis occurs in the majority of cases and is treated in line with metastatic CM.

Anorectal MMM accounts for 0.05% of colorectal and 1% of anal malignancies.[11] Proportionally, however, anal and rectal MMMs constitute 33% and 42% of total MMM cases.

Overall, 60% of anorectal cases are associated with regional lymph node metastasis and a further 30% have distant metastasis at presentation. Surgical intervention is the mainstay of treatment; however, even with an R0 resection the 5 year survival is 19%.[12] The literature suggests there is no benefit of abdominoperineal resection over wide local excision in terms of OS or disease recurrence.[13]

What is the role of ICPIs in MMM?

There has been very little published data on the systemic treatment of MMM, predominantly owing to its rarity and the consequently low numbers of patients enrolled in clinical trials. To date there have been no published randomized controlled trials specifically investigating the use of ICPIs in MMM. A retrospective review of patients receiving ipilimumab revealed that of 33 patients with MMM of any site only a minority gained benefit from treatment:[14] one patient achieved a complete response, one a partial response and six had stable disease; 22 patients had progressive disease and three patients' outcomes were not clear.

A pooled analysis by D'Angelo et al.,[15] in which 10% of trial participants with MMM received either nivolumab monotherapy or ipilimumab and nivolumab in combination, gave insight into the response of MMM in a large group of patients. In the monotherapy setting, there was an overall response rate of 23.3% in patients with MMM, compared with 40.9% in patients with CM, and progression-free survival (PFS) of 3 vs 6.2 months. In the combination setting, the overall response rate was 37.1% vs 60.4%, respectively, and PFS 5.9 vs 11.7 months. Grades 3–4 irAEs were slightly lower in patients with MMM than in patients with CM: respectively, 8.1% vs 12.5% in the monotherapy setting and 40.0% vs 54.9% in the combination setting.[15]

These retrospective reviews[14,15] suggest that ICPIs have activity in MMM (as reflected in the present case report), albeit probably lower than that observed in CM. There are currently insufficient patient numbers to compare outcomes in different subtypes of MMM.

Other options for treatment in MMM include targeted therapy, with up to 10% of cases having a BRAF V600 mutation and a further 25% having a KIT mutation.[16] Serine/threonine-protein kinase B-Raf (BRAF) inhibitors are indicated in patients with a BRAF mutation. In the KIT mutation-positive population a series of phase II trials with imatinib have shown potential benefit in those with exon 11 and exon 13 mutations; however, the relevance of c-KIT amplification in those without a mutation is unclear.[17]

Chemotherapy appears to have a limited role in line with the efficacy in CM. Although limited, the evidence in chemotherapy suggests that there is a median OS of 10.3 months and an overall response rate of 10% in single-agent therapy and 8% in combination therapy.[18]

What endocrinopathies can be caused by ICPIs?

Oncological ICPI therapies evoke adverse inflammatory and autoimmune complications known as irAEs. Endocrinopathies including hypophysitis, hypopituitarism, hypoadrenalism, thyroiditis and type 1 diabetes have all been reported as irAEs secondary to ICPI therapies (Figure 7.1, Table 7.2).[19] They are particularly relevant as they are commonly associated with irreversible loss of endocrine function and require long-term hormone replacement. While in some cases patients present with overt clinical symptoms of endocrinopathies it is very common for patients to be asymptomatic or describe non-specific, nebulous symptoms. Generally symptoms are easily managed with hormone replacement and patients do not usually have to discontinue ICPI treatment.[20] The European Society for Medical Oncology (ESMO) guidelines state that ICPIs should be withheld until symptoms have resolved, after which ICPI treatment may recommence.[21]

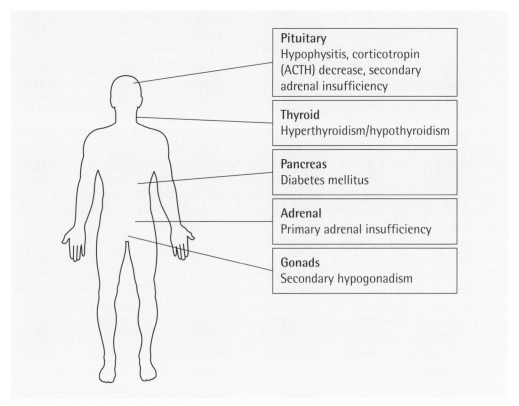

Figure 7.1 Distribution of endocrinopathies.

Table 7.2 Incidence (%) of endocrinopathies with ICPIs (adapted from Sznol *et al.*[19]).

Endocrinopathy	Pembrolizumab		Nivolumab		Ipilimumab and nivolumab	
	Any	Grades 3–4	Any	Grades 3–4	Any	Grades 3–4
Any event	NR	NR	14.4	0.6	30.0	4.8
Hypophysitis	0.7	0.4	0.6	0.3	7.7	1.6
Primary adrenal insufficiency	NR	NR	0.6	0.3	2.6	1.6
Secondary adrenal insufficiency	NR	NR	0.0	0.0	0.3	0.0
Hyperthyroidism	3.2	0.0	4.2	0.0	9.9	1.0
Hypothyroidism	8.7	0.0	8.6	0.0	15.0	0.3
Diabetes mellitus	0.4	0.4	0.0	0.0	0.3	0.0

NR, not reported.

What is the recommended management of diabetes secondary to ICPI therapy?

The development of diabetes mellitus associated with ICPI therapy may take a number of forms. Overall, *de novo* diabetes occurs in less than 1% of patients on mono- or combination therapy.[18] The incidence appears highest with PD-1 blockade, as does that of the other endocrinopathies. While frank diabetic ketoacidosis certainly occurs, patients may also develop a more gradual reduction in glycaemic control that may be managed on oral glucose-lowering drugs and may not require insulin. Additionally, patients may develop impaired glycaemic control secondary to extensive use of high-dose steroids to treat other irAEs.[20] The ESMO guidelines recommend that blood glucose is regularly monitored throughout treatment to detect the emergence of diabetes.[21] The Society for Endocrinology guidelines state that diabetic ketoacidosis and hyperglycaemic hyperosmolar state should be managed as per local guidance.[20] Both guidelines suggest measurement of C-peptide and glutamic acid decarboxylase antibodies. Following stabilization in the acute setting, patients should be referred to local endocrinology or diabetes services for ongoing management of glycaemic control. If a patient is on a reducing course of corticosteroids, the glucose-lowering medication should be titrated accordingly over the weaning period.

Conclusion and learning points

- MMM is a rare and aggressive form of melanoma predominantly affecting the epithelial lining of the head and neck along with the gastrointestinal and genitourinary tracts.

- MMM commonly recurs despite optimal surgical resection and radiotherapy. Local recurrence is often associated with distant metastasis.

- Inoperable and recurrent disease may be treated with radiotherapy, but there is an increasing role for systemic therapies.

- ICPIs have shown promise in MMM. Despite response and outcome data suggesting a lower benefit compared with CM, the (albeit) limited data available show significant benefit from ICPIs, which was also illustrated by the case presented here.

- Endocrine irAEs are common with ICPI therapy and are generally irreversible, requiring long-term hormone replacement.

- Diabetes is a serious side effect of ICPIs and patients may present in diabetic ketoacidosis. Some patients develop *de novo* diabetes, requiring long-term glycaemic management. Others require monitoring and interventions to manage blood glucose while on corticosteroids, which resolves on completion of steroid therapy.

References

1   Chang AE, Karnell LH, Menck HR. The National Cancer Data Base report on cutaneous and noncutaneous melanoma: a summary of 84,836 cases from the past decade. The American College of Surgeons Commission on Cancer and the American Cancer Society. *Cancer* 1998; 83: 1664–78.

2   Meleti M, Leemans CR, de Breer R, *et al*. Head and neck mucosal melanoma: experience with 42 patients, with emphasis on the role of postoperative radiotherapy. *Head Neck* 2008; 30: 1543–51.

3 Pandey M, Mathew A, Abraham EK, *et al*. Primary malignant melanoma of the mucous membranes. *Eur J Surg Oncol* 1998; 24: 303–7.

4 Carvajal RD, Spencer SA, Lydiatt W. Mucosal melanoma: a clinically and biologically unique disease entity. *J Natl Compr Canc Netw* 2012; 10: 345–56.

5 Pfister DG, Ang KK, Brizel DM, *et al*. Mucosal melanoma of the head and neck. *J Natl Compr Canc Netw* 2012; 10: 320–38.

6 Nandaphalan V, Roland NJ, Helliwell TR, *et al*. Mucosal melanoma of the head and neck. *Clin Otolaryngol Allied Sci* 1998; 23: 107–16.

7 Patel SG, Prasad ML, Escrig M, *et al*. Primary mucosal malignant melanoma of the head and neck. *Head Neck* 2002; 24: 247–57.

8 Lee SP, Shimizu KT, Tran LM, *et al*. Mucosal melanoma of the head and neck: the impact of local control on survival. *Laryngoscope* 1994; 104: 121–6.

9 Canavan TP, Cohen D. Vulvar cancer. *Am Fam Physician* 2002; 66: 1269–74.

10 Wechter ME, Gruber SB, Haefner HK, *et al*. Vulvar melanoma: a report of 20 cases and review of the literature. *J Am Acad Dermatol* 2004; 50: 554–62.

11 Cagir B, Whiteford MH, Topham A, *et al*. Changing epidemiology of anorectal melanoma. *Dis Colon Rectum* 1999; 42: 1203–8.

12 Nilsson PJ, Ragnarsson-Olding BK. Importance of clear resection margins in anorectal malignant melanoma. *Br J Surg* 2010; 97: 98–103.

13 Droesch JT, Flum DR, Mann GN. Wide local excision or abdominoperineal resection as the initial treatment for anorectal melanoma? *Am J Surg* 2005; 189: 446–9.

14 Postow MA, Luke JJ, Bluth MJ, *et al*. Ipilimumab for patients with advanced mucosal melanoma. *Oncologist* 2013; 18: 726–32.

15 D'Angelo SP, Larkin J, Sosman JA, *et al*. Efficacy and safety of nivolumab alone or in combination with ipilimumab in patients with mucosal melanoma: a pooled analysis. *J Clin Oncol* 2017; 35: 226–35.

16 Zebary A, Jangard M, Omholt K, *et al*. *KIT, NRAS* and *BRAF* mutations in sinonasal mucosal melanoma: a study of 56 cases. *Br J Cancer* 2013; 109: 559–64.

17 Carvajal RD, Antonescu CR, Wolchok JD, *et al*. KIT as a therapeutic target in metastatic melanoma. *JAMA* 2011; 305: 2327–34.

18 Shoushtari AN, Bluth MJ, Goldman DA, *et al*. Clinical features and response to systemic therapy in a historical cohort of advanced or unresectable mucosal melanoma. *Melanoma Res* 2017; 27: 57–64.

19 Sznol M, Postow MA, Davies MJ, *et al*. Endocrine-related adverse events associated with immune checkpoint blockade and expert insights on their management. *Cancer Treat Rev* 2017; 58: 70–6.

20 Higham C, Olsson-Brown A, Larkin J, *et al*. Society for Endocrinology endocrine emergency guidance: acute management of the endocrine complications of checkpoint inhibitor therapy. *Endocr Connect* 2018; 7: G1–7.

21 Haanen JBAG, Carbonnel F, Robert C, *et al*. Management of toxicities from immunotherapy: ESMO clinical practice guidelines for diagnosis, treatment and follow-up. *Ann Oncol* 2017; 28 (suppl 4): iv119–42.

08 Adjuvant Immunotherapy in Metastatic Melanoma

Helen Adderley, Avinash Gupta

Case history

A 51-year-old woman with no significant medical history was diagnosed with stage IIIB (T2aN1aM0) V600D *BRAF*-mutant melanoma in 2012 after excision biopsy of a long-standing upper back lesion. Histology demonstrated a 1.7 mm non-ulcerated malignant melanoma. Wide local excision showed no evidence of residual disease. Sentinel lymph node biopsy identified one lymph node with isolated cells; she declined completion lymphadenectomy. The patient commenced regular ultrasound surveillance with her local team.

Unfortunately, 4 years later she developed a solitary 1.5 cm enlarged right axillary lymph node. Fine needle aspiration confirmed metastatic melanoma. A PET-CT scan excluded disease elsewhere. The patient underwent right axillary lymphadenectomy, which identified one 18 mm lymph node out of 22 replaced by tumour, with no evidence of extracapsular spread. She was then enrolled on to KEYNOTE-054, a randomized double-blind phase III study of adjuvant pembrolizumab vs placebo in resected high-risk melanoma.

After cycle 4 of treatment she developed grade 2 diarrhoea. Treatment was interrupted and a weaning regimen of oral prednisolone was commenced. After 12 weeks the diarrhoea resolved and study treatment was resumed. Symptoms recurred, however, after cycle 7. Treatment was stopped for a second time and a flexible sigmoidoscopy was done. Mild patchy erythema was seen and biopsies showed features in keeping with immunotherapy-associated colitis. Owing to recurrent toxicity the patient was taken off study in April 2017, oral steroids were adjusted and sulfasalazine was added. Later that month the patient was admitted to hospital with possible pneumonitis, adrenal insufficiency and sepsis, which were managed with steroid adjustment and antibiotics. Diarrhoea fluctuated over the course of 2017, and a further full colonoscopy performed in June 2017 identified similar features in keeping with immunotherapy-associated colitis. Gradually her symptoms settled and prednisolone was slowly weaned down.

Despite multiple immunotherapy-related toxicities, the patient made a full recovery and additional immunosuppression was not required. Steroids were discontinued in January 2018 and she remains disease-free with no evidence of metastatic disease to date.

What is the evidence for adjuvant immunotherapy in melanoma?

Which patients should be selected for adjuvant immunotherapy?

Was the decision to decline initial completion lymphadenectomy correct?

What are the patient's treatment options at relapse?

What is the evidence for adjuvant immunotherapy in melanoma?

Immunotherapy targeting programmed cell death protein 1 (PD-1) and cytotoxic T lympho-cyte-associated protein 4 (CTLA-4) has been firmly established in patients with advanced mela-noma.[1,2] In more recent years the role of adjuvant immunotherapy in patients with completely resected high-risk stage III or IV disease has been explored, with positive results reported by three major randomized controlled trials (RCTs): Efficacy Study of Ipilimumab versus Placebo to Prevent Recurrence after Complete Resection of High Risk Stage III Melanoma (EORTC 18071);[3] Efficacy Study of Nivolumab Compared to Ipilimumab in Prevention of Recurrence of Melanoma after Complete Resection of Stage IIIB/C or Stage IV Melanoma (CheckMate 238);[4] and Study of Pembrolizumab (MK-3475) versus Placebo after Complete Resection of High-Risk Stage III Melanoma (KEYNOTE-054).[5] An Investigational Immunotherapy Study of Nivolumab Combined with Ipilimumab Compared to Nivolumab by Itself after Complete Surgical Removal of Stage IIIB/C/D or Stage IV Melanoma (CheckMate 915) is an ongoing phase III trial (esti-mated primary completion date 2020). In the UK, adjuvant immunotherapy is currently only available through clinical trials. The results of these studies are, however, likely to change the way in which melanoma is treated in the future. Adjuvant treatment is currently being evaluated by NICE.

EORTC 18071

This double-blind international phase III RCT of adjuvant ipilimumab vs placebo after complete resection of high-risk stage III melanoma assigned 951 patients 1:1 to receive ipilimumab 10 mg/kg or placebo every 3 weeks for four doses, then every 3 months for up to 3 years. All patients recruited between 2008 and 2011 were included in the intention-to-treat analysis. Me-dian recurrence-free survival was 26.1 months (95% CI 19.3, 39.3) in the ipilimumab group vs 17.1 months (95% CI 13.4, 21.6) in the placebo group (HR 0.75; 95% CI 0.64, 0.9; $p=0.0013$). Grades 3–5 immune-related adverse events were 43% in the ipilimumab arm vs 2% in the pla-cebo arm.

CheckMate 238

This double-blind international phase III RCT of adjuvant nivolumab vs ipilimumab in resected stage IIIB/IIIC/IV melanoma recruited 906 patients in 2015 and assigned them 1:1 to receive nivolumab 3 mg/kg 2 weekly or ipilimumab 10 mg/kg 3 weekly for four doses and then 12 week-ly for up to 1 year. The 12 month rate of recurrence-free survival was 70.5% in the nivolumab group (95% CI 66.1%, 74.5%) vs 60.8% in the ipilimumab group (95% CI 56.0%, 65.2%). The HR for disease recurrence or death significantly favoured nivolumab (HR 0.65; 97.56% CI 0.51, 0.83; $p<0.001$). Lower rates of grades 3 and 4 toxicity were also demonstrated in the nivolumab arm (14.4% vs 45.9%).

KEYNOTE-054

This double-blind international phase III RCT of adjuvant pembrolizumab vs placebo in resected stage IIIA (>1 mm metastasis), IIIB and IIIC melanoma assigned 1019 patients 1:1 to receive either pembrolizumab 200 mg 3 weekly or placebo for up to 1 year. The 12 month recurrence-free survival rate was 75.4% in the pembrolizumab group vs 61% in the placebo group (HR for disease recurrence or death 0.57; 98.4% CI 0.43, 0.74; $p<0.001$). The rate of grades 3–5 adverse events was 14.7% with pembrolizumab vs 3.4% in the placebo arm.

Which patients should be selected for adjuvant immunotherapy?

Data from the three major trials detailed above highlight the benefit of adjuvant immunotherapy in completely resected stage IIIB/IIIC/IV disease. KEYNOTE-054 also included those with stage IIIA disease with metastasis measuring >1 mm; while there was evidence of benefit in this sub-group, the numbers were small and did not reach statistical significance. High-risk node-negative patients (stage IIB/IIC) were excluded from these trials, so at present there is no evidence to support adjuvant therapy in stage IIB or IIC melanoma. Further clinical trials of adjuvant treatment in this patient population are, however, planned.

Was the decision to decline initial completion lymphadenectomy correct?

Sentinel lymph node biopsy is associated with increased melanoma-specific survival among those with node-positive intermediate thickness melanomas (defined as 1.2–3.5 mm). The value of completion lymphadenectomy in patients with sentinel node involvement was unclear until the recent Multicenter Selective Lymphadenectomy Trial II (MSLT-II).[6] This international phase III RCT examined melanoma-specific survival after completion dissection or observation follow-up in patients with sentinel node-positive melanoma who were randomly assigned 1:1 to upfront completion lymph node dissection or nodal observation. The trial did not meet its primary end-point, as immediate completion lymph node dissection was not associated with increased melanoma-specific survival among the 1934 patients analysed in the intention-to-treat population or in the 1755 patients in the per protocol analysis. In the per protocol analysis the mean 3 year rate of melanoma-specific survival was 86±1.3% in the dissection group vs 86±1.2% in the observation group ($p=0.42$), at a median follow-up of 43 months. Disease-free survival was slightly higher in the dissection group at 3 years because of the increased rate of disease control in regional nodes. The rate of lymphoedema was 24.1% in the dissection group vs 6.3% in the observation group. Based on these results our patient's decision to decline initial lymphadenectomy would not have had a significant impact on relapse and would have potentially avoided unnecessary morbidity.

What are the patient's treatment options at relapse?

As the patient had a V600D *BRAF* mutation she would be eligible for targeted therapy: either serine/threonine-protein kinase B-Raf (BRAF) inhibitor monotherapy or combination BRAF plus mitogen-activated protein kinase kinase (MEK) inhibitor treatment.[7] BRAF and MEK inhibitors work by targeting the mitogen-activated protein kinase (MAPK) pathway and would be suitable treatment options at relapse. Further immunotherapy would also be possible, with ipilimumab plus nivolumab available on the NHS as first line treatment for metastatic disease via the Blueteq registration system (i.e. patients treated with adjuvant immunotherapy are not excluded). It would be important, however, to consider potential risks of toxicity given the patient's previous complications, plus the likely effectiveness, depending on the time to relapse.

Conclusion and learning points

- There is strong evidence from multiple phase III RCTs to support the use of adjuvant immunotherapy in resected stage III or IV melanoma.

- Adjuvant combination immunotherapy is currently being evaluated in a phase III RCT; results are eagerly awaited.

- Adjuvant ipilimumab and nivolumab are approved as monotherapy by the US Food and Drug Administration, and are currently undergoing evaluation by the European Medicines Agency and NICE.

- Completion lymphadenectomy after a positive sentinel lymph node biopsy does not improve overall survival and may be associated with increased morbidity.

- At relapse, further treatment would potentially include further immunotherapy or targeted therapy with BRAF or BRAF plus MEK inhibitors.

- Previous immunotherapy-related toxicity should inform decisions about treatment options at relapse.

References

1   National Institute for Health and Care Excellence (2016). *Nivolumab in combination with ipilimumab for treating advanced melanoma. Technical appraisal guidance TA400.* Available from www.nice.org.uk/guidance/ta400 (accessed 24 April 2018).

2   Larkin J, Chiarion-Sileni V, González R, *et al.* Combined nivolumab and ipilimumab or monotherapy in untreated melanoma. *N Engl J Med* 2015; 373: 23–34.

3   Eggermont AMM, Chiarion-Sileni V, Grob JJ, *et al.* Adjuvant ipilimumab versus placebo after complete resection of high risk stage III melanoma (EORTC 18071): a randomised, double-blind, phase 3 trial. *Lancet Oncol* 2015; 16: 522–30.

4   Weber J, Mandala M, Del Vecchio M, *et al.* Adjuvant nivolumab versus ipilimumab in resected stage III or IV melanoma. *N Engl J Med* 2017; 377: 1824–35.

5   Eggermont AMM, Blank CU, Mandala M, *et al.* Adjuvant pembrolizumab versus placebo in resected stage III melanoma. *N Engl J Med* 2018; 378: 1789–801.

6   Faries MB, Thompson JF, Cochran AJ, *et al.* Completion dissection or observation for sentinel-node metastasis in melanoma. *N Engl J Med* 2017; 376: 2211–22.

7   National Institute for Health and Care Excellence (2016). *Trametinib in combination with dabrafenib for treating unresectable or metastatic melanoma. Technology appraisal guidance TA396.* Available from www.nice.org.uk/guidance/ta396 (accessed 24 April 2018).

Further reading

- American Joint Committee on Cancer. *AJCC cancer staging system.* 8th ed. Available from: https://cancerstaging.org/About/news/Documents/NCRA%20AJCC%20Cancer%20 Staging%20Manual%208th%20Edition%20Update.pdf (accessed 24 April 2018).

- Fife BT, Bluestone JA. Control of peripheral T-cell tolerance and autoimmunity via the CTLA-4 and PD-1 pathways. *Immunol Rev* 2008; 224: 166–82.

- Graziani, G, Tentori, L, Navarra, P. Ipilimumab: a novel immunostimulatory monoclonal antibody for the treatment of cancer. *Pharmacol Res* 2012; 65: 9–22.

- National institute for Health and Care Excellence (2015). *Melanoma assessment and management. Clinical guideline NG14.* Available from www.nice.org.uk/guidance/ng14 (accessed 24 April 2018).

- NHS England (2017). *National cancer drugs fund list.* Available from: www.england.nhs.uk/publication/national-cancer-drugs-fund-list (accessed 13 June 2018).

- Pardoll DM. The blockade of immune checkpoints in cancer immunotherapy. *Nat Rev Cancer* 2012; 12: 252–64.

- Rudd CE, Taylor A, Schneider H. CD28 and CTLA-4 coreceptor expression and signal transduction. *Immunol Rev* 2009; 229: 12–26.

09 Ongoing Response after Stopping Immunotherapy

Zena Salih, Avinash Gupta

Case history

An 81-year-old man with a history of malignant melanoma excised from his left posterior shoulder 17 years ago presented with a new subcutaneous lesion in the left axilla, which was fully resected. Histology confirmed in-transit metastasis and therefore stage IIIB disease. His medical history included hypertension, hypercholesterolaemia, atrial fibrillation and a previous stroke. Medications comprised atorvastatin, bisoprolol and dabigatran.

Three months later, he had an asymptomatic relapse with a solitary right infrahilar node on routine 'high-risk' imaging surveillance. A biopsy showed *BRAF* wild-type metastatic melanoma; a PET-CT scan was recommended by the multidisciplinary team to ascertain the need for surgical resection. Unfortunately, the scan showed stage IV disease with multiple metastases in the left femur, C4 vertebral body and duodenum. The patient decided to proceed with immunotherapy and consented to single-agent pembrolizumab after detailed discussions regarding risks, benefits and his personal goals of treatment.

After cycle 1 of pembrolizumab in January 2016, he had an asymptomatic grade 2 transaminitis; as both alanine aminotransferase (ALT) and aspartate aminotransferase (AST) were three times the upper limit of normal (ULN), cycle 2 was deferred. He was advised to discontinue atorvastatin and an urgent full liver screen was undertaken. He returned 72 h later for clinic review. Hepatitis serology, autoantibody screen, iron studies and liver ultrasound were unremarkable. He had now, however, developed a grade 2 erythematous rash affecting both forearms and worsening grade 3 transaminitis; ALT and AST were 7 × ULN. Oral prednisolone 1 mg/kg per day was therefore commenced.

Two days later, he was hospitalized due to concerns that his liver function tests were slow to improve despite oral corticosteroids. He was then escalated to intravenous methylprednisolone 1 mg/kg per day. Within 5 days, his liver function tests had normalized and the rash had fully resolved. He was discharged home on a reducing course of oral prednisolone.

The patient was monitored weekly as an outpatient and came off prednisolone 8 weeks later. His liver function tests remained normal. A restaging CT scan 3 months after starting immunotherapy revealed a complete radiological response with no measurable disease. Given his significant immune-related hepatotoxicity following one dose of pembrolizumab it was decided not to recommence it. He continues on active surveillance; at last follow-up, 18 months since treatment discontinuation, he remains in remission.

When do immune-related adverse events (irAEs) occur?

What is the evidence for clinical outcome in patients who discontinue treatment early due to toxicity?

Is there any evidence that toxicity is associated with efficacy, and does immuno-suppression with steroids and/or steroid-sparing agents to treat irAEs reduce the anti-tumour efficacy of immune checkpoint blockade?

In the absence of toxicity, what is the evidence for optimal duration of treatment?

When do irAEs occur?

In general, with programmed cell death protein 1 (PD-1)/programmed death-ligand 1 (PD-L1) blockade, irAEs tend to occur within the first few weeks to 3 months after starting treatment. Some toxicities seem to emerge earlier in the course of treatment, but most irAEs are not expected to develop within the first 4 weeks of treatment. There appears to be a pattern of development of the different immune toxicities, with skin and gastrointestinal toxicity generally occurring in the first 4–6 weeks, whereas liver and endocrine manifestations tend to occur later, usually after 3 months.[1]

irAEs may, however, develop at any time, even after discontinuation of treatment, and may wax and wane over time. It has been noted that in some cases the initial onset of irAEs has been as long as 1 year after treatment cessation. While anti-PD-1 or anti-PD-L1 therapy may be used for months and even years, most studies have indicated that extended treatment does not result in a higher cumulative incidence of irAEs.[2]

irAEs associated with the cytotoxic T lymphocyte-associated protein 4 (CTLA-4) inhibitor ipilimumab may occur at any point, but usually present after the third or fourth dose. They are often mild to moderate, but occur in approximately 60–85% of patients. Toxicities directly correlate with ipilimumab dose; the incidence of grade 3 or higher is approximately 10–27%.[3]

irAEs have been observed in 95% of patients receiving combination immunotherapy treatment with ipilimumab and nivolumab. In 55% of patients these were of grade 3 or higher.[4]

The onset of grades 3–4 toxicities for monotherapy with nivolumab or combination immunotherapy differs, as irAEs may not only develop earlier in combination therapy (for example skin toxicity may occur within 24 h of the first dose) but may also develop over a prolonged period of time.[3]

Before starting treatment with immune checkpoint inhibitors (ICPIs), patients should be assessed specifically for their susceptibility to developing irAEs. Some may be at higher risk of irAEs, e.g. those with underlying autoimmune disease. As such patients were excluded from clinical trials, the safety of ICPIs in this group is less clear. Retrospective studies have indicated that immune checkpoint blockade is safe and effective in patients with underlying autoimmune conditions. While these patients may be at risk of transient exacerbation of their autoimmune condition, as well as irAEs, they have largely not been high-grade toxic effects. Patients with an underlying autoimmune disorder should be considered for treatment with immune checkpoint blockade, but caution regarding risks and benefits of treatment should be encouraged.[5] Similarly, patients who have had irAEs on ipilimumab are at risk of developing irAEs after subsequent anti-PD-1 treatment and vice versa.[3]

The risk of toxicity from immune checkpoint blockade, several years after the initiation of treatment, remains unknown. This issue will become progressively more pertinent as indications for immunotherapy treatment extend to patients with cancer at earlier stages, when life expectancy is measured in decades.[5]

What is the evidence for clinical outcome in patients who discontinue treatment early due to toxicity?

A pooled analysis of randomized phase II and III trials was carried out to investigate the impact on outcomes of early discontinuation. It showed that patients with advanced melanoma who discontinued combination immunotherapy because of adverse events did just as well as those who continued treatment uninterrupted.[6] The objective response rate was not just similar in the discontinuation group but numerically higher (58.3% vs 50.2%). Median overall survival (OS) has not yet been reached in either group but thus far is not significantly different in the follow-up ($p=0.23$).[6]

The efficacy of nivolumab plus ipilimumab seemed to be similar in those who continued treatment and in those who discontinued treatment because of irAEs.[6] This suggests that patients may continue to derive benefit from combination therapy even after treatment is stopped due to adverse events. These data contribute to growing doubts about the benefit of extended treatment.[7]

Is there any evidence that toxicity is associated with efficacy, and does immunosuppression with steroids and/or steroid-sparing agents to treat irAEs reduce the anti-tumour efficacy of immune checkpoint blockade?

Some studies suggest that patients with irAEs have higher response rates compared with those who do not experience toxicity; however, this is yet to be fully validated. Indeed, in a large retrospective study of ipilimumab, treatment outcomes were similar in patients with and without irAEs.[8] The overall impression is that toxicity is not required to yield benefit from ICPIs.

It is proposed that specific irAEs are more directly linked to anti-tumour response than others. For example, multiple studies in melanoma patients have shown links between vitiligo and positive clinical outcomes.[9,10] As vitiligo is a side effect that is directly related to antigen-specific immunity, it may be more strongly correlated with anti-tumour efficacy compared with other irAEs.

It is also important to consider whether immunosuppression with steroids and/or steroid-sparing agents to treat irAEs reduces the anti-tumour efficacy of immune checkpoint blockade. Although there are no prospective studies testing immunosuppressive strategies to address this, retrospective studies have indicated that, overall, outcomes are not inferior in patients who receive immunomodulatory agents to manage ICPI-related toxicities compared with outcomes in patients who do not.[8,11] There could be distinct exceptions to this, possibly associated specifically with the type of immunosuppressive treatment used.[12]

In the absence of toxicity, what is the evidence for optimal duration of treatment?

ICPIs are an established standard of care for metastatic melanoma, but there is no definitive information about how long to treat in the absence of toxicity. There is emerging evidence to suggest that many patients may be treated for too long.

There are ongoing efforts to formulate recommendations for duration of treatment, but these are being pursued without the benefit of the blinded and controlled studies required to provide definitive guidance. In the published controlled trials, various schedules have been examined with different ICPIs or combination therapies over different time periods. In the initial phase III ipilimumab trial, treatment was given for only 3 months.[13] In the phase III pembrolizumab trial, treatment was intended for 2 years.[14] In two phase III trials with nivolumab, no limit was placed on treatment duration beyond disease progression.[15]

While complete responses were reached with ICPI therapy in all of these studies, it is uncertain whether length of treatment played a role in protection from relapse when an objective response was attained. The question remains whether further treatment is advantageous once patients achieve a complete response.

Follow-up in the phase IB KEYNOTE-001 trial with pembrolizumab suggests that extended benefit is achieved after a relatively short period of treatment.[16] Sixty-seven patients stopped pembrolizumab after achieving a complete response following at least 6 months of therapy. Of the 67 patients, 61 (91%) remain in complete response after a median follow-up exceeding 3 years. Of the six patients no longer in complete response, two died of other causes, leaving only four patients (6%) who have so far progressed after achieving a complete response. All four were re-treated, but a partial response was achieved in only one patient and there were no complete responses. We cannot draw conclusions about re-challenge from this small number of patients, but it appears that complete response is durable with 3 years of follow-up in the majority of patients included in this *post hoc* analysis.[16]

These data suggest that most patients stay in remission for extended or indefinite periods after achieving a complete response. Stopping an ICPI after a partial response or stable disease is more difficult. KEYNOTE-006, a study evaluating the safety and efficacy of two different dosing schedules of pembrolizumab compared with ipilimumab in patients with advanced melanoma, explores this issue further, with 104 responders discontinuing pembrolizumab after 2 years of treatment.[17] This group included 24 patients with a complete response, 68 with a partial response and 12 with stable disease. Although the median follow-up since stopping the ICPI is only 9.7 months, progression has only been seen in one patient with a complete response, in four with a partial response and in two with stable disease. This is encouraging, as the progression-free survival curves indicate that 91% of patients have maintained benefit despite having stopped the drug.

Definitive information on stopping ICPIs is important because these drugs are expensive and they are associated with a significant burden of adverse events. In the absence of objective evidence, best practice for stopping ICPIs remains unknown. A randomized trial for discontinuing therapy is the only way in which to obtain level 1 evidence to guide clinical practice. In the UK, the forthcoming DANTE study (EudraCT 2017–002435–42) will seek to address this issue. In this phase III trial, patients who have not progressed after 12 months of first line pembrolizumab or nivolumab monotherapy will be randomized either to continue treatment until progression or to stop treatment with the option to resume it on progression if it is felt to be appropriate.

Conclusion and learning points

- irAEs may occur at any time, even after discontinuation of treatment.
- The response rate, depth of response and OS do not seem to be reduced in patients who discontinue treatment because of irAEs.
- The merits and optimal duration of ongoing anti-PD-1 therapy after discontinuation because of irAEs will require prospective evaluation.
- The predictive utility of early-onset irAEs also requires further study.

- There is no validated evidence to suggest that patients who experience toxicity have higher response rates to immune checkpoint blockade.

- There is no evidence that the clinical outcome of patients on ICPIs is affected by the use of immunosuppressive agents for the management of immune-related toxicities.

- There is currently no definitive information on how long to continue treatment with immune checkpoint blockade in the absence of toxicity. A prospective clinical trial to evaluate this will help to guide best practice.

References

1 Postow MA. Managing immune checkpoint-blocking antibody side effects. *Am Soc Clin Oncol Educ Book* 2015; 1: 76–83.

2 Topalian SL, Sznol M, McDermott DF, *et al*. Survival, durable tumor remission, and long-term safety in patients with advanced melanoma receiving nivolumab. *J Clin Oncol* 2014; 32: 1020–30.

3 Haanen JBAG, Carbonnel F, Robert C, *et al*. Management of toxicities from immunotherapy: ESMO clinical practice guidelines for diagnosis, treatment and follow-up. *Ann Oncol* 2017; 28 (suppl 4): iv119–42.

4 Larkin J, Chiarion-Sileni V, González R, *et al*. Combined nivolumab and ipilimumab or monotherapy in untreated melanoma. *N Engl J Med* 2015; 373: 23–34.

5 Postow MA, Sidlow R, Hellman MD. Immune-related adverse events associated with immune checkpoint blockade. *N Engl J Med* 2018; 378: 158–68.

6 Schadendorf D, Wolchok J, Hodi S, *et al*. Efficacy and safety outcomes for patients with advanced melanoma who discontinued treatment with nivolumab and ipilimumab because of adverse events; a pooled analysis of randomized phase II and phase III trials. *J Clin Oncol* 2017; 35: 3807–14.

7 Wolchok J, Chiarion-Sileni V, González R, *et al*. Overall survival with combined nivolumab and ipilimumab in advanced melanoma. *N Engl J Med* 2017; 377: 1345–56.

8 Horvat TZ, Adel NG, Dang TO, *et al*. Immune-related adverse events, need for systemic immunosuppression, and effects on survival and time to treatment failure in patients with melanoma treated with ipilimumab at Memorial Sloan Kettering Cancer Center. *J Clin Oncol* 2015; 33: 3193–8.

9 Hua C, Boussemart L, Mateus C, *et al*. Association of vitiligo with tumor response in patients with metastatic melanoma treated with pembrolizumab. *JAMA Dermatol* 2016; 152: 45–51.

10 Teulings HE, Limpens J, Jansen SN, *et al*. Vitiligo-like depigmentation in patients with stage III–IV melanoma receiving immunotherapy and its association with survival: a systematic review and meta-analysis. *J Clin Oncol* 2015; 33: 773–81.

11 Weber JS, Hodi FS, Wolchok JD, *et al*. Safety profile of nivolumab monotherapy: a pooled analysis of patients with advanced melanoma. *J Clin Oncol* 2017; 35: 785–92.

12 Esfahani K, Miller WH Jr. Reversal of autoimmune toxicity and loss of tumor response by interleukin-17 blockade. *N Engl J Med* 2017; 376: 1989–91.

13 Hodi FS, O'Day SJ, McDermott DF, *et al*. Improved survival with ipilimumab in patients with metastatic melanoma. *N Engl J Med* 2010; 363: 711–23.

14 Robert C, Schachter J, Long GV, *et al*. Pembrolizumab versus ipilimumab in advanced melanoma. *N Engl J Med* 2015; 372: 2521–32.

15 Long GV, Weber JS, Larkin J, *et al.* Nivolumab for patients with advanced melanoma treated beyond progression: analysis of 2 phase 3 clinical trials. *JAMA Oncol* 2017; 3: 1511–19.

16 Robert C, Ribas A, Hamid O, *et al.* Durable complete response after discontinuation of pembrolizumab in patients with metastatic melanoma. *J Clin Oncol* 2018; 36: 1668–74.

17 Schachter J, Ribas A, Long GV, *et al.* Pembrolizumab versus ipilimumab for advanced melanoma: final overall survival results of a multicentre, randomised, open-label phase 3 study (KEYNOTE-006). *Lancet* 2017; 390: 1853–62.

10 Pneumonitis after Treatment with an Anti-PD-1 Antibody in a Patient with Non-Small-Cell Lung Carcinoma

Claire Storey, Anna Beattie, Alastair Greystoke

Case history

A 65-year-old man presented with a 6 week history of cough, fatigue, progressive breathlessness and significant weight loss. He had a 5 pack-year smoking history and had been a non-smoker since his 20s. He had no significant medical history and up to this point had been fit and well. Eastern Cooperative Oncology Group performance status was 0–1 and Medical Research Council dyspnoea score was 2.

Chest X-ray showed meniscal opacification at the left base (Figure 10.1). A subsequent CT scan demonstrated a left-sided pleural effusion with smooth pleural enhancement and a small peripheral pulmonary nodule. Small bilateral lung nodules were noted, and the possibility of early lymphangitis was raised (Figure 10.2). Video-assisted thoracoscopy pleural biopsy revealed a stage IV *TTF1*-positive lung adenocarcinoma.

Gene profiling demonstrated no evidence of *ALK* translocation or *EGFR* mutation. Programmed death-ligand 1 (PD-L1) staining was seen in 100% of the tumour cells at immunohistochemistry.

The patient was initiated on first line pembrolizumab. After three cycles, restaging CT showed improvement of the pleural thickening but progressive ground glass changes and pulmonary nodularity. A diagnosis of grade 1 pneumonitis was made and pembrolizumab was withheld.

The patient was re-challenged with pembrolizumab 6 weeks later but after two further treatments he presented acutely with increasing breathlessness and hypoxia. He was diagnosed with worsening grade 2 pneumonitis (Figure 10.3, chest X-ray; Figure 10.4, CT scan), which was treated promptly by cessation of pembrolizumab and initiation of high-dose oral steroids (1 mg/kg per day). This caused resolution of some of the CT changes and the patient improved clinically.

Given the severity of his pneumonitis, pembrolizumab was permanently discontinued and cancer therapy was changed to cisplatin and pemetrexed chemotherapy. Oral steroids were weaned.

What is the evidence supporting pembrolizumab use in this setting?

What is the differential diagnosis?

How should the patient be investigated?

Does the radiology support the diagnosis of pneumonitis?

How should the patient be managed?

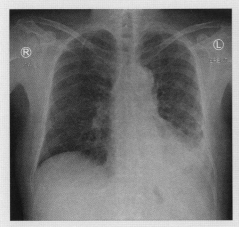

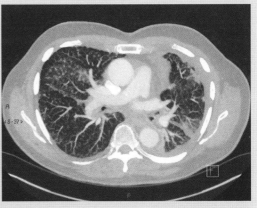

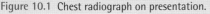

Figure 10.1 Chest radiograph on presentation.

Figure 10.2 Lung windows from staging CT scan
performed at time of diagnosis of stage IV NSCLC.

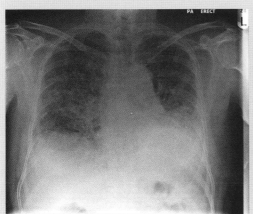

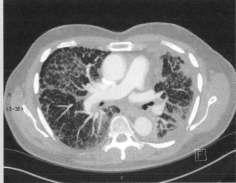

Figure 10.3 Chest radiograph at time of presentation
with acute dyspnoea following re-challenge with
pembrolizumab.

Figure 10.4 Lung windows from urgent CT
pulmonary angiogram at time of presentation
with acute dyspnoea following re-challenge with
pembrolizumab.

What is the evidence supporting pembrolizumab use in this setting?

The Study of Pembrolizumab Compared to Platinum-Based Chemotherapies in Participants with
Metastatic Non-Small Cell Lung Cancer (KEYNOTE-024) randomized 305 patients with non-
small-cell lung carcinoma (NSCLC) who had not yet received systemic therapy for advanced
disease, and where >50% of tumour cells on biopsy demonstrated PD-L1 expression (500 [30.2%]
of the 1652 samples tested).[1] Patients were randomized 1:1 to receive either 200 mg pembrolizumab every 21 days for up to 35 cycles or investigator-choice platinum-based doublet chemotherapy.
The objective response rate was higher with pembrolizumab than with platinum-based doublet

chemotherapy (45% vs 28%), and progression-free survival was longer (median 10.3 vs 6 months; HR 0.50; 95% CI 0.37, 0.68).

Patients were able to cross over following disease progression. Updated results showed that 94 of 150 patients treated with platinum-based doublet chemotherapy had subsequently been treated with pembrolizumab or another immune checkpoint inhibitor (ICPI), and two patients were still receiving chemotherapy.[2] Even with this crossover, the study is presently demonstrating a median overall survival benefit of 30.2 vs 14.2 months in the pembrolizumab and platinum-based doublet chemotherapy arms, respectively (HR 0.63; 95% CI 0.47, 0.86).

What is the differential diagnosis?

The main differential diagnosis in these patients is between progressive cancer and drug-related pneumonitis. In this case the evaluation was made more complex by the presence of lymphangitis on the baseline CT scan. Other differentials that should be considered for new or progressive chest symptoms include:

- atypical infections including *Mycoplasma*, mycobacterial infections (both TB and atypical), *Legionella* and *Pneumocystis jirovecii*;

- pulmonary emboli;

- pulmonary oedema;

- sarcoidosis.

The incidence of pneumonitis after treatment with pembrolizumab in KEYNOTE-024 was 5.8%, with 2.6% of patients experiencing grade 3 or 4 toxicity.[1] A meta-analysis suggested rates of approximately 1.1% grades 3–5 pneumonitis with programmed cell death protein 1 (PD-1) inhibitors when assessed across all tumour types.[3] The incidence of dyspnoea may be higher in clinical practice because subjects enrolled in clinical trials have to meet strict inclusion and exclusion criteria and may have better performance status than those in community practice; therefore, patients may suffer from worse symptoms even if the extent of lung inflammation is similar.

The timing of onset of symptoms, 10 weeks after initiation of therapy in this case, may help determine the likely cause. The median onset of pneumonitis was 2.1 months in two studies evaluating nivolumab in patients with melanoma (CheckMate 037[4] and CheckMate 066[5]). In a large multi-centre community practice series of mostly melanoma and NSCLC patients, the median onset of pneumonitis with anti-PD-1/anti-PD-L1 therapies was 4.6 months (range 21 days to 19.2 months).[6]

How should the patient be investigated?

The basis of investigation is primarily to exclude other causes of breathlessness. Blood tests are likely to be non-specific in nature. Sputum culture and sensitivity, potentially followed by bronchoscopy and lavage, may be used to look for evidence of infection, particularly atypical organisms.

Imaging, including high-resolution CT of the chest, may help determine tumour response as well as other parenchymal lung changes. The CT features of tumour, pneumonitis or other lung pathologies may be non-specific and overlap. Lung function tests, including transfer factor of the lung for carbon monoxide, may indicate the extent of functional changes and act as a baseline for follow-up, but may not correlate well with symptoms.

European Society for Medical Oncology (ESMO) guidelines suggest that surgical biopsy may be used if there are concerns about diagnostic uncertainty, but the potential gain from formal confirmation of the diagnosis needs to be set against the dangers of the procedure, particularly in severe pneumonitis.[7] Often a decision is made to treat on a presumptive diagnosis of pneumonitis and then monitor for clinical and radiological improvement.

Does the radiology support the diagnosis of pneumonitis?

Multiple radiological patterns have been described with ICPI pneumonitis. The most common are cryptogenic organizing pneumonia (COP) (particularly in NSCLC) or ground glass opacities; however, non-specific interstitial pneumonia, hypersensitivity pneumonia and acute respiratory distress syndrome have all been encountered.[8] All lobes are commonly involved. Acute respiratory distress syndrome and COP pattern of changes may be associated with higher-grade pneumonitis.

How should the patient be managed?

The management of the patient depends on the severity of the pneumonitis,[7,9] which should be graded according to the Common Terminology Criteria for Adverse Events:

- grade 1: asymptomatic with radiological or clinical observations only;
- grade 2: symptomatic, requiring medical intervention or with impact on instrumental activities of daily living;
- grade 3: severe symptoms, limiting self-care or requiring oxygen;
- grade 4: life-threatening respiratory compromise.

For grade 1 pneumonitis it is reasonable to withhold the anti-PD-1/anti-PD-L1 agent while investigating other causes. If there is no progression of symptoms, further immunotherapy may be considered. In a case series of 12 patients with low-grade pneumonitis and clinical resolution of their symptoms managed in this fashion, three (25%) had recurrence of similar severity.[6]

For higher-grade pneumonitis, early consultation with a respiratory physician is key to excluding other causes and managing respiratory symptoms.

For grade 2 pneumonitis, the ESMO guidelines suggest an initial trial of antibiotics for 48 h if there is concern about infection, followed by oral prednisolone (1 mg/kg per day) if there is no improvement.[7] In the case presented here, where there is a convincing history of pneumonitis, oral prednisolone should be started immediately. In patients who respond promptly to therapy, cautious re-treatment with immunotherapy may be considered following resolution of symptoms and radiological improvement.

Intravenous methylprednisolone (2 mg/kg per day) should be given for grade ≥3 pneumonitis, or for grade 2 pneumonitis that does not improve on oral prednisolone after 48 h. Depending on patient wishes, the underlying physiological reserve and estimated prognosis, escalation to a critical care unit for non-invasive or invasive ventilation should be considered. In patients who develop grade 3 pneumonitis, anti-PD-1/anti-PD-L1 therapy should be permanently discontinued.

Guidelines suggest that in the absence of response to intravenous steroids, infliximab should be used.[7] The reported numbers of patients treated for pneumonitis with infliximab are, however, small and it is not certain whether it is as effective in this setting as for other autoimmune side effects such as colitis.

Steroids should be titrated down over 6–8 weeks if symptoms improve. Titration should be slow because relapse of pneumonitis may occur. Given the prolonged immunosuppression, prophylactic treatment with co-trimoxazole (e.g. 480 mg twice daily, three times a week) to prevent *P. jirovecii* pneumonia should be considered

Risk factors for pneumonitis

The risk factors for development of pneumonitis in patients receiving single-agent anti-PD-1/anti-PD-L1 are uncertain. An initial meta-analysis suggested that patients with NSCLC are at increased risk compared with those with other tumour types,[10] but the findings have not been replicated in subsequent studies.[3] It may be that the increased diagnostic difficulties in patients with NSCLC led to the reported higher incidence. The impact of smoking history on the development of pneumonitis is not yet clear.

Patients who have received previous thoracic radiotherapy seem to be at higher risk, particularly if there is evidence of radiation pneumonitis.[11] In a subgroup analysis of the original phase I study of pembrolizumab, 15 of 24 patients who received radiotherapy to the chest reported respiratory symptoms, which in three (13%) were thought to be related to pembrolizumab.[12] In the Global Study to Assess the Effects of MEDI4736 Following Concurrent Chemoradiation in Patients with Stage III Unresectable Non-Small Cell Lung Cancer (PACIFIC), which investigated the anti-PD-L1 durvalumab in patients completing concurrent chemoradiotherapy for stage III NSCLC, radiation pneumonitis of any grade occurred in 33.9% of patients receiving durvalumab vs 24.8% in the standard arm, with a minimal increase in grade ≥3 pneumonitis (3.4% vs 2.6%).[13]

Conclusion and learning points

- Pembrolizumab has superior outcomes compared with chemotherapy in untreated metastatic NSCLC where the tumour expresses PD-L1 in >50% of cells.

- Pneumonitis is a rare complication of treatment with anti-PD-1/anti-PD-L1 antibodies.

- The differential diagnosis in patients with NSCLC presenting with increased dyspnoea while on treatment with anti-PD-1/anti-PD-L1 antibodies is wide and includes tumour progression and pneumonitis.

- Early involvement of respiratory physicians and radiologists is key in the investigation and management of these patients.

- ESMO guidelines outline appropriate management depending on the severity of pneumonitis.

- Patients with severe or steroid refractory pneumonitis should discontinue treatment with anti-PD-1/anti-PD-L1 antibodies.

References

1 Reck M, Rodríguez-Abreu D, Robinson AG, et al. Pembrolizumab versus chemotherapy for PD-L1-positive non-small-cell lung cancer. *N Engl J Med* 2016; 375: 1823–33.

2 Brahmer J, Rodríguez-Abreu D, Robinson A, et al. OA 17.06 Updated analysis of KEYNOTE-024: pembrolizumab vs platinum-based chemotherapy for advanced NSCLC with PD-L1 TPS ≥50%. *J Thorac Oncol* 2018; 12 (11 suppl 2): S1793–4.

3 Khunger M, Rakshit S, Pasupuleti V, et al. Incidence of pneumonitis with use of programmed death 1 and programmed death-ligand 1 inhibitors in non-small cell lung cancer: a systematic review and meta-analysis of trials. *Chest* 2017; 152: 271–81.

4 Weber JS, D'Angelo SP, Minor D, et al. Nivolumab versus chemotherapy in patients with advanced melanoma who progressed after anti-CTLA-4 treatment (CheckMate 037): a randomised, controlled, open-label, phase 3 trial. *Lancet Oncol* 2015; 16: 375–84.

5 Robert C, Long GV, Brady B, *et al*. Nivolumab in previously untreated melanoma without *BRAF* mutation. *N Engl J Med* 2015; 372: 320–30.

6 Naidoo J, Wang X, Woo KM, *et al*. Pneumonitis in patients treated with anti-programmed death-1/programmed death ligand 1 therapy. *J Clin Oncol* 2017; 35: 709–17.

7 Haanen JBAG, Carbonnel F, Robert C, *et al*. Management of toxicities from immunotherapy: ESMO clinical practice guidelines for diagnosis, treatment and follow-up. *Ann Oncol* 2017; 28 (suppl 4): iv119–42.

8 Nishino M, Ramaiya NH, Awad MM, *et al*. PD-1 inhibitor-related pneumonitis in advanced cancer patients: radiographic patterns and clinical course. *Clin Cancer Res* 2016; 22: 6051–60.

9 Puzanov I, Diab A, Abdallah K, *et al*. Managing toxicities associated with immune checkpoint inhibitors: consensus recommendations from the Society for Immunotherapy of Cancer (SITC) Toxicity Management Working Group. *J Immunother Cancer* 2017; 5: 95.

10 Nishino M, Giobbie-Hurder A, Hatabu H, *et al*. Incidence of programmed cell death 1 inhibitor-related pneumonitis in patients with advanced cancer: a systematic review and meta-analysis. *JAMA Oncol* 2016; 2: 1607–16.

11 Tamiya A, Tamiya M, Nakahama K, *et al*. Correlation of radiation pneumonitis history before nivolumab with onset of interstitial lung disease and progression-free survival of patients with pre-treated advanced non-small cell lung cancer. *Anticancer Res* 2017; 37: 5199–205.

12 Shaverdian N, Lisberg AE, Bornazyan K, *et al*. Previous radiotherapy and the clinical activity and toxicity of pembrolizumab in the treatment of non-small-cell lung cancer: a secondary analysis of the KEYNOTE-001 phase 1 trial. *Lancet Oncol* 2017; 18: 895–903.

13 Antonia SJ, Villegas A, Daniel D, *et al*. Durvalumab after chemoradiotherapy in stage III non-small-cell lung cancer. *N Engl J Med* 2017; 377: 1919–29.

Further reading

• Chuzi S, Tavora F, Cruz M, *et al*. Clinical features, diagnostic challenges, and management strategies in checkpoint inhibitor-related pneumonitis. *Cancer Manag Res* 2017; 9: 207–13.

• Fujimoto D, Kato R, Morimoto T, *et al*. Characteristics and prognostic impact of pneumonitis during systemic anti-cancer therapy in patients with advanced non-small-cell lung cancer. *PLoS One* 2016; 11: e0168465.

11 Colitis after Combination Immunotherapy in a Clinical Study of Small-Cell Lung Cancer

Beth Lambourne, John Reicher, Ally Speight, Alastair Greystoke

Case history

A 57-year-old man with chemotherapy refractory small-cell lung cancer presented acutely 2 weeks after his second treatment with combination immunotherapy (anti-programmed cell death protein 1 [PD-1] and anti-cytotoxic T lymphocyte-associated protein 4 [CTLA-4] antibodies). He had a 2 day history of severe abdominal pain and diarrhoea occurring 3–4 times per day. He was tachycardic with a pulse rate of 115 beats/min and a blood pressure of 180/90 mmHg. On examination he had a distended abdomen with hyperactive bowel sounds but no focal tenderness, guarding or other evidence of peritonism.

Blood tests on admission showed neutrophilia (14.86×10^9/ml), acute renal injury (creatinine 165 µmol/l, from baseline 107 µmol/l), elevated C-reactive protein (CRP, 1162 nmol/l) and lactate (4.1 mmol/l). Blood pH and bicarbonate were within normal limits. He was producing large volume stool (type 7 on Bristol Stool Chart) with no blood, which was negative for *Clostridium difficile* toxin, and subsequently negative on microscopy and culture. CT showed dilated, fluid-filled small bowel, mucosal non-enhancement in a jejunal segment, *Pneumatosis intestinalis* (Figure 11.1A, arrow-heads) and gas in the liver (Figure 11.1A, arrow), consistent with ischaemia.

In the absence of peritonism he was managed non-surgically on the intensive care unit with fluid resuscitation, intravenous methylprednisolone (2 mg/kg per day), antibiotics, and patient-controlled analgesia. His symptoms improved dramatically, with concomitant improvement in his blood tests (although CRP climbed to a maximum of 2276 nmol/l 36 h after admission). Repeat CT after 4 days demonstrated complete resolution of the abnormalities (Figure 11.1B). Given the rapid improvement, the ischaemic changes probably represent transient hypoperfusion from colitis leading to hypovolaemia.

How should this patient be managed and investigated initially?

What is the differential diagnosis?

What is the incidence of colitis on immune checkpoint inhibitor (ICPI) therapy?

What is the role of endoscopy?

How should the severity of colitis be assessed?

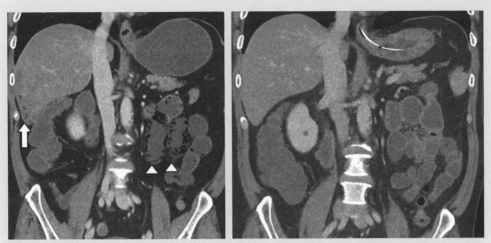

Figure 11.1 (A) CT on admission; (B) CT after 4 days of steroids showing complete resolution of previously seen abnormalities.

How should this patient be managed and investigated initially?

Patients with immunotherapy-related colitis may be very unwell. Initial management should be immediate assessment of the airway, breathing and, in particular, circulation, together with appropriate fluid resuscitation. A full blood count should be performed to look for anaemia and neutrophilia, along with biochemical profiles for renal injury, electrolyte imbalance and any concomitant hepatitis. Of note, 37% of patients receiving combination immunotherapy develop an immune-related adverse event (irAE) affecting more than one organ.[1]

CRP should be assessed, although any elevation may be relatively non-specific in this situation, and amylase also measured because autoimmune pancreatitis may cause similar symptoms and co-present with colitis. If the patient is unwell, elevated lactate suggests poor tissue perfusion, the development of metabolic acidosis or the development of sepsis, potentially resulting from bowel perforation.

Stool should be sent urgently for *C. difficile* toxin testing, with microscopy and culture for viruses, bacterial pathogens and parasites.

For patients with tachycardia, abdominal pain, bloody stool, or in those where there is clinical concern on the basis of history, examination or the blood tests listed above, an urgent CT scan of the abdomen and pelvis should be performed. This may help confirm the diagnosis, determine the amount of bowel involved and reveal any perforation and associated collections.

What is the differential diagnosis?

The main differential is gastrointestinal infection. This includes viruses such as norovirus and cytomegalovirus (CMV), bacterial infections such as *C. difficile*, *Campylobacter* and *Salmonella*, or parasites such as cryptosporidium. In patients with tumours such as melanoma or colorectal cancer, the presence of either primary or metastatic disease in the bowel may cause similar symptoms.

In this case study, the severity of the symptoms and the time of onset after combination immunotherapy are in keeping with an iatrogenic colitis. The median time of onset for gastrointestinal toxicity in patients receiving combination immunotherapy is 7.4 weeks (range 1–48.9 weeks).[1] A recent report of 44 patients with suspected immune-related colitis after treatment with single-agent anti-PD-1/programmed death-ligand 1 (PD-L1) found that only 20 patients had confirmed colitis, whereas 11 had symptoms related to tumour and eight had self-limiting diarrhoea with no obvious abnormality found despite investigation.[2]

What is the incidence of colitis on ICPI therapy?

The incidence of immunotherapy-related colitis depends on the treatment given. It is higher with anti-CTLA-4 antibodies such as ipilimumab than with anti-PD-1/PD-L1 agents such as nivolumab, pembrolizumab and atezolizumab. The incidence is highest with combination immunotherapy.

This was well demonstrated in the phase III CheckMate 067 study in which 945 patients with melanoma were randomized in a double-blind manner 1:1:1 to ipilimumab (3 mg/kg every 21 days in four doses), nivolumab (3 mg/kg every 14 days) or both (ipilimumab 3 mg/kg every 21 days and nivolumab 1 mg/kg for four cycles followed by nivolumab 3 mg/kg every 14 days).[1] In this study the incidence of grade 3 or 4 diarrhoea was 6.1% with ipilimumab, 1.2% with nivolumab and 9.3% with the combination. Any grade colitis was reported in 11.6% with ipilimumab, 1.3% with nivolumab and 11.8% with the combination.

Similarly, a recent systematic review of 34 studies and over 8500 patients found that the incidence of grade 3 or 4 diarrhoea was 7.9% with ipilimumab, 2.2% with nivolumab and 9.2% with the combination. Any grade colitis was reported in 9.1% with ipilimumab, 0.9% with nivolumab and 13.6% with the combination.[3]

What is the role of endoscopy?

Endoscopy is useful in establishing the diagnosis, determining the severity and helping to rule out alternative aetiologies. Even when the colon looks macroscopically normal, systematic biopsies may reveal a clinically significant microscopic colitis.[4] Endoscopic scoring systems established in inflammatory bowel disease, such as the Mayo Endoscopic Score, seem to have limited utility in this setting and correlate poorly with symptoms and outcomes.[4]

Endoscopy may help determine the extent of involvement and whether ulceration is present. Immunotherapy-related colitis may have a patchy colonic distribution, unlike the contiguous inflammation seen in acute, severe ulcerative colitis. Furthermore, patients are more likely to be steroid refractory and require rescue infliximab treatment when more than three segments of bowel are involved and/or where mucosal ulceration is present.[4,5] Superadded CMV colitis has been reported in immunotherapy-related colitis, and the presence of CMV DNA in the biopsy may be associated with steroid refractory disease.[6]

How should the severity of colitis be assessed?

Most guidelines start with grading the diarrhoea according to the Common Terminology Criteria for Adverse Events (CTCAE):[7,8]

- grade 1: increase in <4 stools/day over baseline;
- grade 2: increase in 4–6 stools/day over baseline;
- grade 3: increase in ≥7 stools/day over baseline; incontinence; hospitalization indicated; limiting self-care;
- grade 4: life-threatening consequences; urgent intervention indicated.

It is important to recognize, however, that this assessment of diarrhoea may not accurately determine the severity of the underlying colitis. Warning signs that there may be a potentially severe episode of colitis include tachycardia, abdominal pain and bloody stool.

For grade 1 diarrhoea it is reasonable to treat the patient with loperamide, encourage oral fluids and make dietary adjustments such as omitting or lowering lactose intake (involvement of the small bowel mucosa may lead to decreased lactase manufacture and temporary relative intolerance). Provided symptoms settle quickly, immunotherapy may be continued while other causes for diarrhoea are investigated.

For higher-grade colitis, early consultation with a gastroenterologist is key to help exclude other causes and manage symptoms.

For grade 2 diarrhoea lasting more than 3 days, or where there are additional causes for concern such as tachycardia, abdominal pain or bloody stool, further immunotherapy should be withheld while the patient undergoes investigation. Oral prednisolone (1 mg/kg per day) should be started. If there is no improvement within 72 h, the patient should be treated as for grades 3–4 colitis.

For colitis grade ≥3, or lower-grade colitis not improving on oral prednisolone within 72 h, intravenous methylprednisolone (2 mg/kg per day) is required. Depending on patient wishes, the underlying physiological reserve and estimated prognosis, escalation to a critical care unit for closer monitoring and inotropic support should be considered. If there is no evidence of bowel perforation on CT, and symptoms do not improve within 72 h, or worsen, then the patient should be treated with a single dose of infliximab (5 mg/kg). Infliximab should not be given where there is previous TB, hepatitis B or C, or severe cardiac failure. In one case series, infliximab resolved diarrhoea in a median of 2 days, and 10 out of 12 patients responded to this treatment.[9] A further infliximab treatment may need to be given 2 weeks later and was required in up to 50% of cases in one series.[4]

Occasionally, additional immune suppression may be needed. Agents include mycophenolate mofetil, tacrolimus or the anti-integrin α4β7 antibody vedolizumab which prevents T cells localizing to the intestine.

If there is bowel perforation, a surgical opinion should be urgently sought and consideration given to subtotal colectomy.

Which patients are at risk?

The main risk factor for the development of colitis is the type of immunotherapy, as described above. Patients receiving NSAIDS may also be at higher risk.[9]

Re-treatment in patients who have previously developed colitis with ipilimumab is likely to result in relapse.[9] Although colitis relapse is rare when using an anti-PD-1/PD-L1 agent, rates of other irAEs may be higher, affecting up to 21%, compared with the normal population.[10] Consequently these patients should be monitored closely if immunotherapy re-challenge is undertaken. As a rule, further immunotherapy is contraindicated in patients with severe immune-related gastrointestinal toxicity.

Conclusion and learning points

- Colitis is a relatively common complication of treatment with anti-CTLA-4 antibodies, either as single agent or in combination with anti-PD-1, but is also seen in 1–2% of patients receiving anti-PD-1 alone.
- Early involvement of gastroenterologists and surgeons is key in the investigation and management of these patients.

- While CTCAE grading of diarrhoea is useful in initial assessment of patients, it may not correlate with severity of colitis.
- Tachycardia, abdominal pain or bloody stool should prompt urgent investigation and management.
- Appropriate management depends on the severity of colitis, as outlined in the European Society for Medical Oncology guidelines.
- Patients with severe colitis should discontinue treatment with immunotherapy.

References

1 Larkin J, Chiarion-Sileni V, González R, *et al*. Combined nivolumab and ipilimumab or monotherapy in untreated melanoma. *N Engl J Med* 2015; 373: 23–34.

2 Collins M, Michot JM, Danlos FX, *et al*. Inflammatory gastrointestinal diseases associated with PD-1 blockade antibodies. *Ann Oncol* 2017; 28: 2860–5.

3 Wang DY, Ye F, Zhao S, Johnson DB. Incidence of immune checkpoint inhibitor-related colitis in solid tumor patients: a systematic review and meta-analysis. *Oncoimmunology* 2017; 6: e1344805.

4 Geukes Foppen MH, Rozeman EA, van Wilpe S, *et al*. Immune checkpoint inhibition-related colitis: symptoms, endoscopic features, histology and response to management. *ESMO Open* 2018; 3: e000278–2017–000278.

5 Jain A, Lipson EJ, Sharfman WH, *et al*. Colonic ulcerations may predict steroid-refractory course in patients with ipilimumab-mediated enterocolitis. *World J Gastroenterol* 2017; 23: 2023–8.

6 Franklin C, Rooms I, Fiedler M, *et al*. Cytomegalovirus reactivation in patients with refractory checkpoint inhibitor-induced colitis. *Eur J Cancer* 2017; 86: 248–56.

7 Haanen JBAG, Carbonnel F, Robert C, *et al*. Management of toxicities from immunotherapy: ESMO clinical practice guidelines for diagnosis, treatment and follow-up. *Ann Oncol* 2017; 28 (suppl 4): iv119–42.

8 Puzanov I, Diab A, Abdallah K, *et al*. Managing toxicities associated with immune checkpoint inhibitors: consensus recommendations from the Society for Immunotherapy of Cancer (SITC) Toxicity Management Working Group. *J Immunother Cancer* 2017; 5: 95.

9 Marthey L, Mateus C, Mussini C, *et al*. Cancer immunotherapy with anti-CTLA-4 monoclonal antibodies induces an inflammatory bowel disease. *J Crohn's Colitis* 2016; 10: 395–401.

10 Menzies AM, Johnson DB, Ramanujam S, *et al*. Anti-PD-1 therapy in patients with advanced melanoma and preexisting autoimmune disorders or major toxicity with ipilimumab. *Ann Oncol* 2017; 28: 368–76.

12 Jaundice after Pembrolizumab in a Patient with Melanoma and Brain Metastases

Gary J. Doherty, Pippa G. Corrie

Case history

A 49-year-old woman was admitted to hospital with a 3 week history of morning headaches, followed by a 7 day history of blurred vision and vomiting. Her medical history included surgical excision of a thoracic cutaneous *BRAF*-mutant primary melanoma and axillary lymph node clearance 2 years previously.

A CT scan of the head, chest, abdomen and pelvis, followed by an MRI scan of the head, revealed multiple bilateral cerebral metastases (with surrounding oedema) and multiple small-volume subcutaneous and peritoneal nodules. The patient improved on high-dose oral dexamethasone and received whole brain radiotherapy (20 Gy in five fractions), which resulted in a mixed intracranial response. Her steroids were weaned over the following 2 weeks, after which treatment with intravenous pembrolizumab (2 mg/kg every 3 weeks) was commenced. Her Eastern Cooperative Oncology Group performance status was 1.

Eight days later the patient developed jaundice associated with marked (Common Terminology Criteria for Adverse Events [CTCAE] grade 3) liver function derangement (bilirubin 90 µmol/l, alkaline phosphatase 3.96 µkat/l, gamma-glutamyltransferase 34.97 µkat/l, aspartate aminotransferase 16.05 µkat/l and alanine aminotransferase 25.65 µkat/l), with normal prothrombin time. A liver screen was later confirmed as unremarkable and oral prednisolone (1 mg/kg per day) was commenced.

Liver function continued, however, to worsen (Figure 12.1) and the patient underwent a liver biopsy. Liver histopathology showed an absence of cytokeratin 7 staining (a marker for biliary epithelium), without a significant inflammatory infiltrate. Oral mycophenolate mofetil (1 g twice daily) was added.

Liver function did not improve in the subsequent 2 months, during which the patient developed insulin-dependent diabetes mellitus, a painful thoracic vertebral wedge fracture, profound hypocalcaemia, a rising international normalized ratio (INR) and, later, profound neutropenia.

Three months after her first pembrolizumab dose, restaging CT showed progressive disease in the peritoneum. In the face of abnormal liver blood tests, the patient was commenced on oral dabrafenib at 25% full dose (75 mg once daily) and increased to 50% full dose (75 mg twice daily) after 2 weeks. A partial response in the extracranial disease and a mixed response in the intracranial disease were observed.

Oral trametinib (1 mg once daily) was added, and both trametinib and dabrafenib were cautiously escalated to full treatment doses (2 mg once daily and 150 mg twice daily).

Over the next 8 months, her liver function slowly improved and systemic treatment was well tolerated. The patient ultimately died from progressive intracranial disease 6 months after starting dabrafenib.

Was this patient's treatment sequencing optimal?

What should be performed in a full liver screen, and what is the differential diagnosis for the liver injury in this case?

What is the incidence and nature of T cell immune checkpoint inhibitor (ICPI)-induced hepatotoxicity and what is the optimal management of such cases?

What were the likely causes of the complications seen after starting mycophenolate mofetil and how could these be managed?

Why were the doses of dabrafenib and trametinib escalated so cautiously? Could this patient have been re-challenged with immunotherapy?

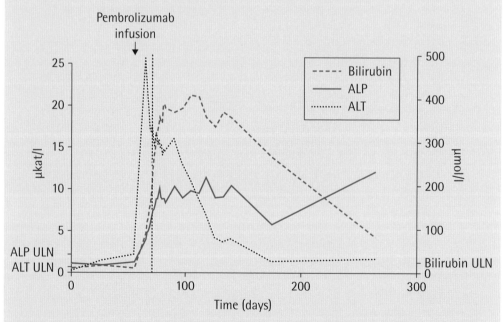

Figure 12.1 Evolution of the patient's liver function tests over time, annotated with the timing of pembrolizumab administration and liver biopsy. ALP, alanine phosphatase; ALT, alanine aminotransferase; ULN, upper limit of normal.

Was this patient's treatment sequencing optimal?

The life-threatening disease at presentation with metastatic melanoma was the extensive, symptomatic intracranial metastatic disease, which was coupled with small-volume extracranial disease. Rapid disease control was only required for the intracranial disease. The high rate of intracranial response to the serine/threonine-protein kinase B-Raf (BRAF) inhibitor dabrafenib (39.2% for treatment-naive patients in a phase II trial[1]) suggests that this would have been the most suitable agent to achieve rapid intracranial disease control. Response rates are likely to be even higher with a combination of BRAF and mitogen-activated protein kinase kinase (MEK) inhibitors.

T cell ICPIs also provide intracranial disease control; however, the intracranial response rate of ~22% for pembrolizumab[2] and the slow time to response (as well as the risk of worsening of intracranial symptoms through inflammatory responses) make it a suboptimal choice in this case. ICPIs may be used in patients with asymptomatic, low-volume brain metastases that do not require steroids. A phase II study reported intracranial response rates (in treatment-naive patients) of 20% for nivolumab alone and 46% for nivolumab combined with ipilimumab, albeit with high rates of grades 3–4 toxicity.[3]

Whole brain radiotherapy does not prolong survival in melanoma patients with brain metastases and should be used cautiously. Stereotactic radiosurgery and neurosurgical resection also have roles in patients with progressive (small-volume) brain metastases with controllable extracranial disease. Stereotactic radiosurgery is commissioned in England for patients with a Karnofsky Performance Score ≥70%, life expectancy >6 months and intracranial disease volume ≤20 cc (and individual lesions must usually be <3 cm in diameter).[4] While some retrospective analyses have reported improved outcomes (and manageable toxicity) with concurrent treatment with radiation and systemic therapy, it remains investigational until prospective data suggest otherwise.

What should be performed in a full liver screen, and what is the differential diagnosis for the liver injury in this case?

Given the many competing aetiologies of acute liver failure, a liver screen should include imaging of the liver and portal systems (to investigate infiltrative or obstructive causes), as well as Doppler analysis (to investigate acute vascular events). Blood should be analysed for infectious (viral hepatitis A/B/C/E, cytomegalovirus, Epstein–Barr virus and adenovirus) and metabolic (alpha$_1$-antitrypsin, caeruloplasmin and haemochromatosis) causes. The screen should include immunological analysis for anti-mitochondrial, anti-nuclear, anti-smooth muscle and anti-liver kidney microsomal antibodies and gamma-globulin levels. Given the absence of prior liver disease, the unremarkable liver screen, and the time of onset of liver failure, pembrolizumab-induced hepatotoxicity was the likely cause.

What is the incidence and nature of T cell ICPI-induced hepatotoxicity and what is the optimal management of such cases?

Published rates of hepatotoxicity from T cell ICPIs vary from study to study but overall occur in ~5–10% of treated patients.[5] A meta-analysis of 17 trials reported an odds ratio for hepatotoxicity of 5.01 and 1.94 for anti-cytotoxic T lymphocyte-associated protein 4 (CTLA-4) and anti-programmed cell death protein 1 (PD-1) agents, respectively.[6] The rate is increased when they are applied in combination (~25–30%).[5]

The aetiology is poorly understood, often mimicking sporadic autoimmune hepatitis but without associated autoantibodies. Pathologically, ipilimumab has been associated with panlobular and zone 3 hepatitis, as well as portal inflammation and cholestasis. Nivolumab has been associated with extrahepatic and intrahepatic biliary injury and T cell infiltration around the Glisson's capsule. Pembrolizumab has been associated with biliary injury and ductopenia, including vanishing bile duct syndrome, which was the diagnosis in this case; these abnormalities appear to be poorly steroid responsive.[7]

While mechanisms of injury clearly vary, European Society for Medical Oncology (ESMO) guidelines dictate that suspected CTCAE grades 3–4 T cell ICPI-induced hepatotoxicity should be managed by ICPI discontinuation and prompt introduction of (methyl)prednisolone (1–2 mg/kg per day).[5] If there is no prompt improvement in liver function within 2–3 days, mycophenolate mofetil should be added (0.5–1.0 g orally, twice daily).

We recommend early involvement of specialist hepatologists in the care of such patients, which is also necessary for steroid refractory cases. Anti-thymocyte globulin may be considered for such cases. Ideally, treatment should be guided by histopathological analysis of a liver biopsy where feasible, in concert with hepatology advice. Ursodeoxycholic acid should be commenced when cholestasis is found, as it may help improve liver function.

What were the likely causes of the complications seen after starting mycophenolate mofetil and how could these be managed?

This patient developed new-onset diabetes mellitus, requiring insulin, as well as an osteoporotic spinal wedge fracture, both of which were side effects of steroid use. All patients who require high-dose steroids should have their blood glucose monitored and be considered for bone prophylaxis. Patients should have regular clinical reviews to check for steroidal side effects; if steroids are not helping to improve liver function, they should be weaned to mitigate toxicity.

Neutropenia is a recognized complication of mycophenolate mofetil; patients on this drug should be frequently monitored with full blood counts and counselled to seek emergency medical help if pyrexia and/or infection develops. The rising INR and hypocalcaemia in this case were accompanied by very low vitamin K and vitamin D levels, a consequence of fat-soluble vitamin malabsorption owing to cholestasis. Both issues responded promptly to exogenous vitamin K and vitamin D.

Why were the doses of dabrafenib and trametinib escalated so cautiously? Could this patient have been re-challenged with immunotherapy?

Both dabrafenib and trametinib undergo hepatic metabolism and biliary excretion, necessitating careful dosing in cases of liver failure, weighing up the intended benefits and considerable attendant risks. We recommend starting at low doses and up-titrating depending on tolerance and clinical/radiological appearances. Given the risk of worsening an already potentially life-threatening toxicity, ESMO guidelines do not recommend re-challenge with immunotherapy in the context of grade 3 or 4 hepatotoxicity.[5]

Conclusion and learning points

- Sequencing metastatic melanoma therapies is not straightforward, but patients with *BRAF*-mutant metastatic melanoma who develop symptomatic and multiple brain metastases will most likely gain more from initiating BRAF-targeted therapy first.
- Hepatotoxicity from T cell ICPIs is increasingly encountered in clinical practice and should be treated promptly with high-dose steroids to prevent life-threatening consequences.

- Immunosuppressive therapies may have significant side effects and should only be used in the longer term if they are likely to be helping to improve liver function.

- Close, active monitoring and supportive care for the consequences of liver injury and the side effects of immunosuppressive medications are warranted in these complex cases.

- Holistic decisions regarding further systemic anticancer treatment should be made by counterbalancing the intended benefits and attendant risks (particularly if metabolized by hepatic/biliary routes).

References

1   Long GV, Trefzer U, Davies MA, *et al.* Dabrafenib in patients with Val600Glu or Val600Lys *BRAF*-mutant melanoma metastatic to the brain (BREAK-MB): a multicentre, open-label, phase 2 trial. *Lancet Oncol* 2012; 13: 1087–95.

2   Goldberg SB, Gettinger SN, Mahajan A, *et al.* Pembrolizumab for patients with melanoma or non-small-cell lung cancer and untreated brain metastases: early analysis of a non-randomised, open-label, phase 2 trial. *Lancet Oncol* 2016; 17: 976–83.

3   Long GV, Atkinson V, Lo S, *et al.* Combination nivolumab and ipilimumab or nivolumab alone in melanoma brain metastases: a multicentre randomised phase 2 study. *Lancet Oncol* 2018; 19: 672–81.

4   NHS Commissioning Board (2013). *Clinical commissioning policy: stereotactic radiosurgery/ radiotherapy for cerebral metastases.* Available from: www.england.nhs.uk/wp-content/ uploads/2013/04/d05-p-d.pdf (accessed 2 February 2018).

5   Haanen JBAG, Carbonnel F, Robert C, *et al.* Management of toxicities from immunotherapy: ESMO clinical practice guidelines for treatment, diagnosis and follow-up. *Ann Oncol* 2017; 28 (suppl 4): iv119–42.

6   Wang W, Lie P, Guo M, *et al.* Risk of hepatotoxicity in cancer patients treated with immune checkpoint inhibitors: a systematic review and meta-analysis of published data. *Int J Cancer* 2017; 141: 1018–28.

7   Doherty GJ, Duckworth AM, Davies SE, *et al.* Severe steroid-resistant anti-PD1 T-cell checkpoint inhibitor-induced hepatotoxicity driven by biliary injury. *ESMO Open* 2017; 2: e000268.

13 Localized Scleroderma in a Patient with Metastatic Melanoma Treated with Pembrolizumab

Claire M. Connell, Sarah J. Welsh, Conor Broderick, Marc Wallace, Pippa G. Corrie

Case history

A 33-year-old woman with a history of a stage IIIB melanoma treated by resection and left axillary dissection 3 years previously was referred to the melanoma oncology clinic with surveillance-detected pulmonary and brain metastases. CT imaging identified multiple bilateral pulmonary metastases (maximum diameter 22 mm). MRI head identified a 13 × 11 mm enhancing lesion at the grey–white matter junction of the right posterior cingulate cortex, with surrounding vasogenic oedema (Figure 13.1A), and a further 8 mm diameter lesion in the right inferior temporal lobe. She was asymptomatic, her performance status was 0, and she had no comorbidities and no regular medications other than an oral contraceptive (ethinylestradiol/drospirenone). Treatment with pembrolizumab was initiated (2 mg/kg, every 3 weeks).

After four cycles of pembrolizumab, a restaging CT scan demonstrated an interval reduction in the pulmonary metastases (maximum diameter from 22 mm to 5 mm), and MRI demonstrated a reduction in the parietal metastasis (maximum diameter from 13 mm to 4 mm) (Figure 13.1B), with the right inferior temporal metastasis no longer visible. After cycle 5, her hair turned white. After cycle 7, she complained of increasing fatigue, which was associated with elevated thyroid-stimulating hormone (120 mIU/l), for which levothyroxine was commenced. From cycle 18, she developed symmetrical depigmentation affecting the back of her hands and neck.

At cycle 20, she developed dry, pruritic and painful tight skin on the lateral aspects of her neck, chest, upper arms and thighs that progressed rapidly and began to limit neck movement. On examination, the skin was shiny, indurated and thickened (Figure 13.1C). In addition, the symmetrical depigmentation began to involve her upper arms and thighs. There was no eye, mouth or genital involvement and no respiratory or gastrointestinal symptoms. Histology from a deep incisional biopsy from her right arm was consistent with a diagnosis of localized scleroderma (also termed morphoea). Autoantibody screen was negative (including double-stranded DNA, centromere, ribosomal P, proliferating cell nuclear antigen [PCNA], ribonucleoprotein [RNP], Sm, Ro, La, Scl-70, Jo-1, polymyositis/scleroderma [PM/Scl], fibrillarin, RNA polymerase III, Mi-2, NOR-90, Th/To and Ku). Spirometry was normal (forced expiratory volume in one second [FEV$_1$]/forced vital capacity [FVC]). The combination of localized scleroderma, xerosis cutis and vitiligo was consistent with immune-related toxicity generated by pembrolizumab.

How would you manage this patient with pembrolizumab-induced localized scleroderma?

What is the evidence base for the treatment of immunotherapy-associated scleroderma?

Does pembrolizumab-associated scleroderma generate the same complications as systemic sclerosis?

Are there any risk factors for pembrolizumab-associated scleroderma?

A   B

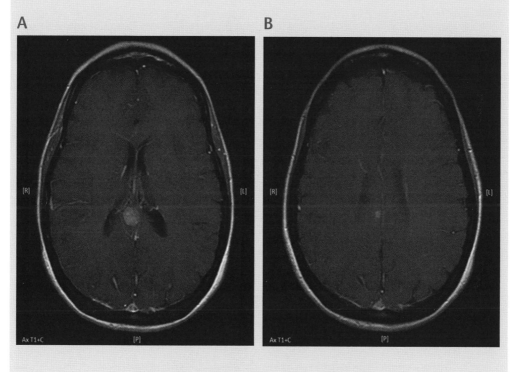

C

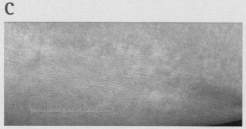

Figure 13.1 (A, B) MR head with contrast demonstrating an enhancing lesion at the grey–white matter junction of the right posterior cingulate cortex at presentation (A) and after four cycles of pembrolizumab (B). (C) Shiny, indurated and thickened skin developing after cycle 20 of pembrolizumab.

How would you manage this patient with pembrolizumab-induced localized scleroderma?

Pembrolizumab was stopped and advice from dermatology specialists was sought. The patient was managed initially with high-dose prednisolone (1 mg/kg once daily, with bone and gastrointestinal tract protection) and, after histological confirmation of scleroderma, was started on hydroxy-chloroquine 200 mg once daily, increased after 1 week to 200 mg twice daily, with a weaning dose of prednisolone (reduced by 5 mg per week). Systemic immunosuppression was supplemented with a topical steroid (mometasone furoate 0.1%, followed by calcipotriol 0.005%/betamethasone dipropionate 0.05% ointment) and regular emollients. After only 2 weeks there was a clinical improvement in her scleroderma, with functional improvement in her neck movement. After 2 months she was started on maintenance methotrexate therapy (5 mg weekly, titrated up by 5 mg a week, with folic acid), hydroxychloroquine was stopped and prednisolone wean was completed.

Within 4 weeks of stopping prednisolone, the patient developed new plaques of morphoea and increased activity in previously quiescent disease. We therefore increased methotrexate to 20 mg weekly and restarted prednisolone. She remained on methotrexate 20 mg weekly and her prednisolone dose was gradually reduced. A restaging CT, 21 months after starting pembrolizumab, demonstrated a complete response and no evidence of malignancy.

What is the evidence base for the treatment of immunotherapy–associated scleroderma?

Although skin is an organ commonly affected by immunotherapy, scleroderma has only rarely been reported, so there are currently no specific guidelines on the optimal management of this specific immune-related adverse event (irAE). Experience from a limited number of case reports[1] must be supplemented by the management principles of scleroderma and immunotherapy-associated toxicities more generally. The consensus advice is to stop pembrolizumab in the presence of severe irAEs and seek early advice from specialist teams. In this case, dermatologists oversaw use of both topical treatment and early systemic immunosuppressive therapy with prednisolone, hydroxy-chloroquine and methotrexate. A similar combination regimen has previously been reported to generate a good clinical response.[1]

Does pembrolizumab–associated scleroderma generate the same complications as systemic sclerosis?

It is unknown whether these patients are at risk of similar organ complications that characterize systemic sclerosis or are at risk of additional immunotherapy-related toxicities. Although there are currently no documented cases of scleroderma-associated renal crisis in this setting, the possibility should be considered, including the attendant risk from steroid therapy. As demonstrated by this case, however, steroid weaning may be problematic. Maintenance immunosuppressants may be introduced in order to allow steroids to be reduced and withdrawn when possible.

Are there any risk factors for pembrolizumab–associated scleroderma?

The very low incidence of pembrolizumab-associated scleroderma poses limitations in identifying relevant risk factors. A personal or family history of autoimmune disorders (including scleroderma) might predict an increased risk of pembrolizumab-associated scleroderma, and taking a full medical history is always important before starting patients on immunotherapy. Neither, however, was present in our case, nor in previously published cases.[1]

Similarly, scleroderma has been associated with somatic gene mutations in cancer tissue that are sufficient to generate a humoral immune response against both normal and mutated peptides, with mutations in the *POLR3A* gene (which encodes the RNA polymerase III subunit RPC1) being the archetypal example.[2] Although these antibodies would be predicted to increase the risk of pembrolizumab-associated scleroderma, neither our case nor the previously published cases[1] was positive for the serology associated with systemic sclerosis (either systemic [anti-centromere] or diffuse [anti-topoisomerase] variants). Our case was also negative for antibodies against RNA polymerase III, which were not tested in the previously published cases.

The key recommendations at present, therefore, are early diagnosis and instigation of immuno-suppressive therapy. Treatment is facilitated by patient education to report new symptoms early, raising awareness of the various manifestations of immunotherapy toxicities, and seeking input from specialist teams to help guide management.

Conclusion and learning points

- Skin-related irAEs associated with immunotherapy are very common. Most are mild and include skin rash, dryness and itching.

- Localized scleroderma (morphoea) is a rare irAE associated with anti-programmed cell death protein 1 (PD-1) antibody therapy, with a wide range of onset (between cycle 5 and cycle 20, from the three case reports to date).

- Pembrolizumab-associated sclerodermoid reactions appear to be responsive to immunosuppressive therapy; early diagnosis is important.

References

1 Barbosa NS, Wetter DA, Wieland CN, *et al.* Scleroderma induced by pembrolizumab: a case series. *Mayo Clin Proc* 2018; 92: 1158–63.

2 Joseph CG, Darrah E, Shah AA, *et al.* Association of the autoimmune disease scleroderma with an immunologic response to cancer. *Science* 2014; 343: 152–7.

14 Intracranial Melanoma Response to Combination Ipilimumab and Nivolumab

Rebecca Johnson, Miranda Payne

Case history

A 65-year-old man was diagnosed with a high-risk cutaneous melanoma (pT4b). Following wide local excision and negative sentinel lymph node biopsy, he continued under surveillance.

Four years later he experienced a seizure. Imaging demonstrated three new cerebral metastases (right occipital lobe, left caudate nucleus and right lentiform nucleus), one pulmonary metastasis and pathological thoracic lymphadenopathy. Biopsy confirmed metastatic melanoma with a *BRAF* V600 mutation.

At his oncology appointment, he was very well (Eastern Cooperative Oncology Group [ECOG] performance status 0). His only medication was lisinopril and levetiracetam. After detailed discussion about treatment options it was decided to initiate first line combination immunotherapy with ipilimumab and nivolumab. The first two cycles were well tolerated, apart from grade 2 dermatoses requiring emollients, antihistamines and topical steroids.

On day 14 of the third cycle, he was admitted with fatigue, anorexia and new diarrhoea (grade 2). Investigations showed a normal white blood cell count, moderately elevated C-reactive protein (CRP) (571 nmol/l) and raised alanine transaminase (grade 1). Imaging was consistent with mild left-sided colitis but also demonstrated a significant tumour response: the pulmonary metastasis had reduced from 23 mm to 14 mm.

He received 4 days of intravenous methylprednisolone; his diarrhoea improved to grade 1 and he was discharged on high-dose oral prednisolone. At review 10 days post-discharge, he reported that he continued to have his bowels open three to four times a day (grade 1) but bowel function was solely at night. He also described abdominal pain and anorexia and felt generally unwell. Blood tests revealed rising CRP and falling albumin levels. Flexible sigmoidoscopy (day 30 of cycle 3) showed widespread erythema and apthous ulceration.

He was readmitted shortly afterwards with nausea, vomiting and weight loss. White blood cells remained within the normal range and CRP was only moderately elevated (476 nmol/l). He received an infusion of the anti-tumour necrosis factor (TNF) antibody infliximab and demonstrated rapid clinical improvement: within 24 h his nausea had resolved; within 48 h his bowel habit was improving and within 4 days it had returned to baseline.

Four months after starting treatment, imaging showed an excellent response to treatment: the lung metastasis had reduced to 7 mm and subcarinal lymphadenopathy had resolved. Furthermore, there was partial response in the three cerebral metastases, with complete resolution of all perilesional oedema and no new lesions.

How is immunotherapy-related diarrhoea graded? How is it managed?

How effective is immunotherapy in metastatic melanoma without brain metastases?

What is the current approach to management of a patient with melanoma brain metastasis?

What evidence base is there for combination immunotherapy in patients with melanoma brain metastases?

How is immunotherapy–related diarrhoea graded? How is it managed?

In general, immune-related adverse events (irAEs) are graded in terms of severity using the Common Terminology Criteria for Adverse Events on a scale of 1–5, with 1 representing mild cases, and 5 equating to death-related to toxicity.

Grade 1 diarrhoea is defined as an increase in stool frequency of two to three per day and is often managed conservatively. Grade 2 diarrhoea is defined as an increase of four to six stools per day above baseline. Grade 3 diarrhoea is an increase of seven stools per day above baseline (or incontinence), while grade 4 is any life-threatening complication (e.g. intestinal obstruction or perforation), for which all patients should be closely observed. Grading of diarrhoea may, however, be misleading and there is increasing evidence it may not reflect the severity of underlying bowel inflammation, as in the case described above. Direct visualization by colonoscopy or flexible sigmoidoscopy should be undertaken in all patients with grades 3 or 4, or persistent grade 2, diarrhoea but may also provide a more accurate estimate of clinical risk in patients with less severe diarrhoea. All diarrhoea should be treated as grade 3 or 4 if CRP is ≥285 nmol/l and previously within normal limits, haemoglobin or albumin levels are falling when previously normal or, importantly, if symptoms worsen or persist despite more than 7 days' treatment with steroids. Management should also routinely include the exclusion of viral and bacterial infective causes.

Immunotherapy-related diarrhoea is managed by interrupting treatment with immune checkpoint inhibitors and initiating treatment with steroids. For patients with grade 2 diarrhoea, oral prednisolone is often sufficient and is usually commenced at a dose of 60 mg once daily. For patients with more severe diarrhoea, or with other worrying clinical features, intravenous high-dose glucocorticoids (usually methylprednisolone 1 mg/kg once daily) should be initiated. Patients usually benefit from joint management with a gastroenterologist with expertise in immunotherapy-related toxicity. Most patients will improve within 72 h and may be converted to oral prednisolone after a few days, which is gradually reduced usually over at least 6 weeks depending on the response. If no improvement occurs after 3–5 days of intravenous glucocorticoid treatment, escalation to other forms of immunosuppression should be considered. Most commonly this is with the anti-TNF antibody infliximab. Unless there is a prompt response to initial treatment, the patient will be facing prolonged exposure to steroids and consideration should be given to blood glucose monitoring, appropriate bone protection and prophylaxis against *Pneumocystis jirovecii*.

How effective is immunotherapy in metastatic melanoma without brain metastases?

A large-scale randomized phase III clinical trial recently reported by Wolchok *et al.*[1] analysed overall survival (OS) of combined nivolumab and ipilimumab treatment in patients with stage III or intravenous melanoma. All study participants had previously untreated, histologically confirmed disease and a known *BRAF* V600 mutation status. One important exclusion criterion was the presence of intracranial metastases; all participants had an ECOG performance status of 0 or 1.

The trial was run across 21 countries and recruited just under 1300 patients, 945 of whom were randomized 1:1:1 to one of three cohorts and stratified according to programmed death-ligand 1 (PD-L1) status, serine/threonine-protein kinase B-Raf (BRAF) status and metastasis stage. The first cohort received nivolumab plus ipilimumab followed by maintenance nivolumab, the second cohort received nivolumab plus placebo, and the third cohort received ipilimumab plus placebo.

The minimum follow-up time for all surviving patients was 36 months. The study had two primary endpoints: progression-free survival (PFS) and OS. The median PFS was just under 12 months for nivolumab plus ipilimumab, just under 7 months for nivolumab plus placebo, and just under 3 months for ipilimumab plus placebo. Combination therapy of nivolumab and ipilimumab resulted in significantly longer OS at 3 years compared with single-agent therapy with nivolumab or ipilimumab (58% vs 52% and 34%, respectively)

The overall conclusions drawn from the trial were that treatment with anti-programmed cell death protein 1 (PD-1) therapy achieves survival outcomes superior to those with ipilimumab treatment, and that, in turn, combination treatment with nivolumab and ipilimumab produces greater survival benefit compared with nivolumab monotherapy.[1]

What is the current approach to management of a patient with melanoma brain metastasis?

Melanoma is the third most common systemic cancer leading to brain metastases. Melanoma has a predilection for metastasis to the brain: cerebral involvement is found in 20–25% of patients with stage IV melanoma. Furthermore, brain metastases are found in 50–75% of patients at autopsy.[2]

To date, the majority of clinical trials for melanoma have specifically excluded patients with brain metastases. As a result the optimum treatment for such patients remains unknown. Management of brain metastatic melanoma has therefore traditionally focused on symptom control as opposed to active management of the disease. Consequently, most evidence regarding active treatment options for brain metastasis has thus far has relied on individual case reports.

A literature search reveals that, until very recently, active management of brain metastases generally focused on local treatment. Traditional cytotoxic agents do not generally penetrate the blood–brain barrier well, and agents that do, for example temozolomide, have low activity against melanoma. For solitary lesions, the general approach is surgical resection followed by radiotherapy, and for multiple cranial metastases, both stereotactic radiosurgery and whole brain radiotherapy are considered approaches. Unfortunately, however, melanoma has inherent radioresistance.[3]

There have been individual case reports of ipilimumab controlling extracranial disease in patients who have then undergone subsequent local irradiation to control their brain metastasis. A retrospective study of 58 patients with limited brain metastasis who underwent stereotactic radiosurgery investigated the efficacy of additional ipilimumab. Unfortunately, the addition of ipilimumab did not demonstrate improved intracerebral disease control.[4]

A US study enrolled 72 patients with brain metastatic melanoma (cohort A comprised 51 neurologically asymptomatic individuals who were not receiving corticosteroid treatment at study entry; cohort B comprised 21 symptomatic individuals on a stable dose of corticosteroids). Both cohorts were administered 10 mg/kg intravenous ipilimumab every 3 weeks for four doses.[5] After 12 weeks, nine patients in cohort A showed disease control (18%; 95% CI 8%, 31%), as did one patient in cohort B (5%; 95% CI 0.1% to 24%). When the brain alone was assessed, 12 patients in cohort A (24%; 95% CI 13%, 38%) and two in cohort B (10%; 95% CI 1%, 30%) achieved disease control. The most common grade 3 irAEs were diarrhoea, rash and raised liver transaminases. One patient in cohort A died of drug-related complications of immune-related colitis.

In patients with brain metastases with *BRAF*-mutated melanoma, BRAF-targeted treatments have shown significant intracranial responses.[6] Benefit, however, is relatively short lived, as resistance mechanisms occur in the tumours. The longer-term survival documented with immunotherapy is generally not seen; hence, for patients with low-volume asymptomatic *BRAF*-mutant disease or those with *BRAF* wild-type melanoma, immunotherapy remains a reasonable option.

What evidence base is there for combination immunotherapy in patients with melanoma brain metastases?

Recent advances in the development of immunotherapies have led to the availability of novel agents for melanoma patients. Excitingly, and pertinent to this case, a recent phase II clinical trial in Australia (the Anti-PD-1 Brain Collaboration [ABC]), achieved an intracranial response rate of 42% in asymptomatic patients with known melanoma brain metastases who had not previously undergone any local therapy to the brain.

The ABC trial included 76 patients with at least one melanoma brain metastasis of between 5 mm and 40 mm who had had no previous treatment with anti-cytotoxic T lymphocyte-associated protein 4 (CTLA-4), anti-PD-1 or PD-L1 agents. Importantly, patients were not excluded based on any previous exposure to BRAF or mitogen-activated protein kinase kinase (MEK) inhibitors. Furthermore, patients had ECOG performance status 0, 1 or 2 and had no medical history of serious autoimmune diseases or corticosteroid therapy.[7] The study allocated participants to one of three cohorts based on whether they were symptomatic or had received any prior brain radiotherapy.

Patients who were asymptomatic with no previous local brain treatment were randomized into two cohorts. The first cohort received nivolumab plus ipilimumab for four cycles followed by nivolumab monotherapy. The second cohort received nivolumab alone. A third cohort comprising patients who were symptomatic, had known leptomeningeal disease with MRI evidence of progression, or had previously undergone brain radiotherapy received nivolumab alone. At the time of the data cut-off point, 67 of the 76 patients initially recruited had more than 18 weeks' follow-up; their results formed the findings of the study. The range of follow-up times was 5–34 months, with a median of 16.4 months.

The primary endpoint was intracranial response at or after 12 weeks; all results were based on best intracranial response according to the Response Evaluation Criteria in Solid Tumors. Remarkably, there was an intracranial response of 42% for patients receiving nivolumab and ipilimumab, with 15% showing a complete response. This compared with a 20% intracranial response and a 12% complete response in patients who received nivolumab alone. Encouragingly, for all patients who had a complete response, at the point of result publication, not one had progressed.

An intracranial response was seen in 6% of patients in the third cohort who were symptomatic of their disease, had undergone previous cranial irradiation or had progressive leptominingeal disease and had received single-agent nivolumab.[7]

Conclusion and learning points

- Combination immunotherapy with nivolumab and ipilimumab may have excellent results on both cerebral and extracerebral melanoma metastases.
- Grading of gastrointestinal symptoms may be misleading: patients with symptoms persisting for 7 days or more, or who do not respond to steroid therapy, should be managed according to higher severity treatment algorithms.

References

1 Wolchok JD, Chiarion-Sileni V, González R, *et al*. Overall survival with combined nivolumab and ipilimumab in advanced melanoma. *N Engl J Med* 2017; 377: 1345–56.

2 Davies MA, Liu P, McIntyre S, *et al*. Prognostic factors for survival in melanoma patients with brain metastases. *Cancer* 2011; 117: 1687–96.

3 Chukwueke U, Batchelor T, Brastianos P. Management of brain metastases in patients with melanoma. *J Oncol Pract* 2016; 12: 536–42.

4 Mathew M, Tam M, Ott PA, *et al*. Ipilimumab in melanoma with limited brain metastases treated with stereotactic radiosurgery. *Melanoma Res* 2013; 23: 191–5.

5 Margolin K, Ernstoff MS, Hamid O, *et al*. Ipilimumab in patients with melanoma and brain metastases: an open-label, phase 2 trial. *Lancet Oncol* 2012; 13: 459–65.

6 Long GV, Trefzer U, Davies MA, *et al*. Dabrafenib in patients with Val600Glu or Val600Lys *BRAF*-mutant melanoma metastatic to the brain (BREAK-MB): a multicentre, open-label, phase 2 trial. *Lancet Oncol* 2012; 13: 1087–95.

7 Long GV, Atkinson V, Lo S, *et al*. Combination nivolumab and ipilimumab or nivolumab alone in melanoma brain metastases: a multicentre randomised phase 2 study. *Lancet Oncol* 2018; 19: 672–81.

15 Delayed Response to Immunotherapy in a Patient with Acral Melanoma

Benjamin Pickwell-Smith, Ruth E. Board

Case history

A 62-year-old man was diagnosed with a 2.4 mm ulcerated acral lentiginous malignant melanoma of the right great toe nail bed in May 2014. His medical history included essential hypertension, although he was not on any regular medication. He was active and had a performance status of 0. The melanoma was surgically resected by amputation of his right great toe. Sentinel lymph node biopsy was positive: two out of two nodes sampled contained melanoma. He underwent right groin completion lymph node dissection; 12 nodes were removed, one of which contained malignant melanoma. Overall his disease was staged as IIIC malignant melanoma (T3bN2M0). *BRAF* mutation testing was negative. Following multidisciplinary team review he began high-risk follow-up with both oncology and plastic surgery teams.

Two years later a PET-CT scan demonstrated asymptomatic recurrent disease in his right internal and external iliac nodes. These were resected laparoscopically; histological examination showed that 13 out of 19 lymph nodes contained metastatic melanoma.

Three months later he presented with left-sided inguinal lymphadenopathy. A staging CT scan showed a 2 × 1.5 cm left inguinal lymph node but no other areas of metastatic disease. He agreed to start combination immunotherapy with nivolumab and ipilimumab in September 2016. By November 2016 he had completed four cycles, complicated by hypopituitarism treated with hydrocortisone replacement.

A restaging CT scan after four cycles of treatment demonstrated progressive disease with left inguinal lymphadenopathy measuring 3.6 × 2.3 cm, a new pulmonary nodule measuring 5 mm and new mediastinal lymphadenopathy measuring up to 1.9 cm. He remained well, with a performance status of 0, and was referred for consideration of participation in a clinical trial. While going through clinical trial screening it was discovered that his tumour was *KIT* wild-type, prompting further reassessment scans.

A restaging CT scan 8 weeks after stopping treatment showed a delayed response to immunotherapy with a marked regression in the mediastinal lymph nodes but an increase in size of the left inguinal lymph node to 5.4 × 3.4 cm. Several weeks later he observed a spontaneous clinical regression of his left inguinal lymph node. He began maintenance nivolumab therapy. Recent scans show an ongoing response to treatment; on clinical review there was no palpable lymphadenopathy. He remains on nivolumab immunotherapy and hormone replacement therapy; no further toxicities have been observed.

What is the evidence for the treatment of acral melanoma with immunotherapy?

Are there other cases displaying a delayed response to immunotherapy described in the literature?

What are the immune-related response criteria?

What is the evidence for the treatment of acral melanoma with immunotherapy?

Acral lentiginous melanoma occurs on non-hair-containing surfaces of the body such as the palms, soles and under the nails. It is less common in people with lighter skin types. Acral melanomas are morphologically and epidemiologically distinct from non-acral cutaneous melanoma (CM).[1] A small subset of patients with acral melanoma have activating mutations in the *KIT* oncogene and some of these mutations are sensitive to inhibition with tyrosine kinase inhibitors. Research in this area is active in clinical trials.[2] Acral melanomas have a lower somatic mutational burden and poorer prognosis than CM.[3,4] Owing to the rarity of acral melanomas, clinical trials historically do not separately report outcomes for acral melanomas, and it had been hypothesized the efficacy of the immunotherapy agents would be lower in this subtype due to the lower mutational burden. A retrospective multicentre cohort study of advanced or unresectable acral melanoma showed evidence of clinical response to the programmed cell death protein 1 (PD-1) inhibitors pembrolizumab and nivolumab.[5] In a largely second line setting this study reported an objective response rate of 32% (95% CI 15%, 54%) in patients with acral melanoma and a median progression-free survival (PFS) of 4.1 months, thus supporting the use of PD-1 inhibitors in this rarer melanoma subtype.

A retrospective study from two large academic melanoma centres reviewed the clinical outcomes of 35 patients with acral melanoma treated with ipilimumab.[6] The objective response rate was 11.4% and the clinical benefit rate was 22.9% (complete response, partial response or stable disease); median PFS was 2.5 months (95% CI 2.3, 2.7 months). These results are comparable to those in unselected populations.

Are there other cases displaying a delayed response to immunotherapy described in the literature?

There is substantial evidence in the literature of a small percentage of patients on immunotherapy treatment who exhibit a reduction in tumour burden after initial tumour progression. This phenomenon is described in melanoma but is also observed in other solid tumours treated with immunotherapy.[7] One particular study describes four patterns of response in patients with melanoma treated with the anti-cytotoxic T lymphocyte-associated protein 4 (CTLA-4) monoclonal antibody ipilimumab (Figure 15.1).[8]

It is thought that early progressive disease on restaging scans, described as pseudo-progression, is caused by an influx of immune cells following reactivation of the immune response to the tumour, causing a transient increase in tumour burden.[9] In one study, patients treated with ipilimumab who experienced an initial increase in tumour size had repeat biopsies which confirmed inflammatory cell infiltrates or necrosis, and some patients exhibited a later decrease in tumour burden.[10] A further immune-related response pattern also observed in clinical trials of ipilimumab is the development of new lesions. These are associated with oedema and infiltration of immune cells and transient increases in baseline tumour lesions.[8] Delayed clinical responses have

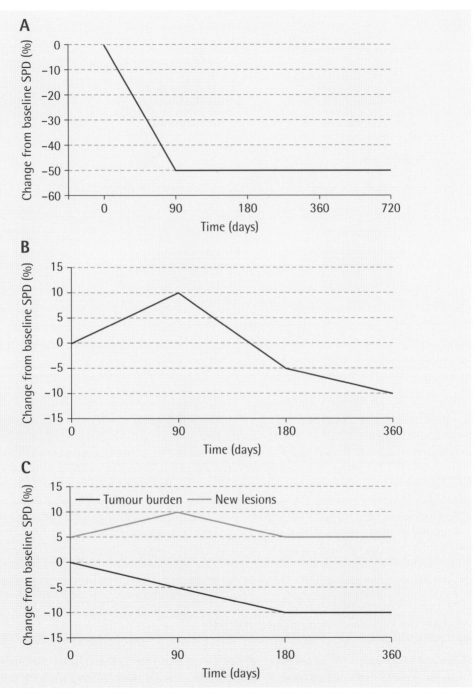

Figure 15.1 Potential patterns of response to immunotherapy: the x-axis is the relative day from the randomization date; the y-axis is the change in tumour volume from baseline. This is shown as the percentage change from baseline in the sum of the product of perpendicular diameters (SPD). (A) Reduction in baseline lesions. (B) Initial increase in tumour burden followed by response. (C) Response in target lesions in the presence of new disease elsewhere.

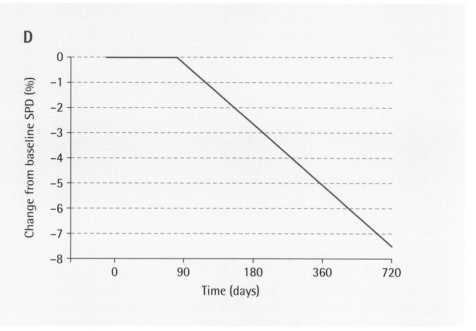

Figure 15.1 (Continued) (D) Stable, durable disease (sometimes with slowly decreasing lesions thereafter). The figures are a representative illustration only and are not based on patient data.

also been observed in studies of other immunotherapeutic agents, in which an initial increase in total tumour burden was later followed by tumour regression.[11] A clinical trial of the anti-PD-1 inhibitor pembrolizumab found that 3.6% of patients met the Response Evaluation Criteria in Solid Tumors (RECIST) for progressive disease at first assessment, followed by a clinical response at second assessment.[11] As experience has increased in treating melanoma with immunotherapies, the observation that some patients may survive for extended periods of time with stable disease as the best objective response supports the hypothesis of immune surveillance as a desirable outcome.[12]

A pooled analysis of trials demonstrated that 95 of 500 patients (19%) in a treatment beyond progression cohort (vs discontinuation at RECIST-defined progressive disease) later had a 30% or greater decrease in tumour burden. Median overall survival in patients with RECIST-defined progressive disease given an anti-PD-1 antibody was longer in the treatment beyond progression cohort compared with the discontinuation at initial sign of progressive disease cohort (Figure 15.2).[11]

What are the immune-related response criteria?

RECIST were developed to standardize the characterization of tumours to chemotherapeutic agents and have become the standard of radiological reporting for treatment responses in clinical trials. With the advent of immunotherapy and targeted therapy there is, however, some concern about using traditional response criteria to determine treatment efficacy. Stable disease, partial response and complete response may all occur after an initial increase in tumour burden on radiological imaging during immunotherapy treatment.[8,13] As such, a novel approach to restaging disease responding to immunotherapy is required. Using RECIST was shown to underestimate

A

B

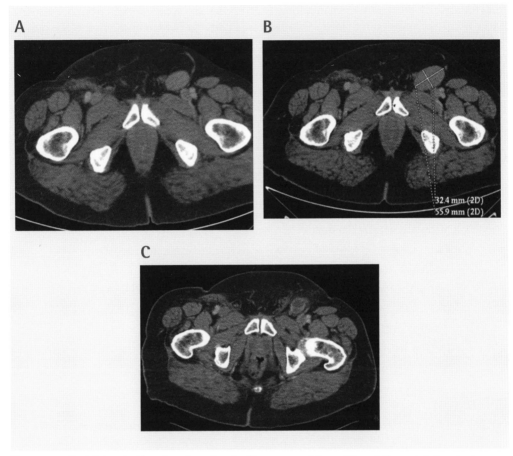

C

32.4 mm (2D)
55.9 mm (2D)

Figure 15.2 The left inguinal lymph node as described in our case at three different time points in order to illustrate our patient's response to immunotherapy. (A) CT scan at baseline prior to systemic therapy. (B) CT scan showing the same lymph node demonstrating pseudo-progression after four doses of ipilimumab and nivolumab. (C) CT scan of the same lymph node showing delayed regression.

the benefit of immunotherapy in approximately 10% of patients in a study designed to compare RECIST with proposed 'immune RECIST'.[11] Multiple other studies have observed distinct immune responses across different solid tumours. Current expert opinion is that immune agents impact host anti-tumour response and may require additional time to achieve measurable or sustained clinical effects compared with traditional chemotherapies.[13]

Therefore, while RECIST 1.1 continues to remain the gold standard for evaluating treatment response in solid tumours to cytotoxic chemotherapy, inaccurate interpretation of response to immunotherapy may result in premature termination of therapy and subsequent removal of patients from clinical trials. The consensus guideline immune-based RECIST (iRECIST) was developed by the RECIST working group in cancer immunotherapy trials.[14] The guideline standardizes and validates immune response criteria accounting for the novel response patterns seen with immunotherapies. The principles used to establish objective tumour response are largely unchanged from RECIST 1.1, but the major change for iRECIST is the concept of redefining tumour response if RECIST 1.1 progression is followed by a decrease in tumour burden by the time of the next assessment.[14] iRECIST uses the term iUPD to denote unconfirmed progressive disease and iCPD for confirmed progressive disease. iUPD requires confirmation by observing a further increase in size (or in the number of new lesions) in the lesion category in which progression was first identified, or progression in lesion categories not previously meeting RECIST 1.1 progression criteria. If no change in tumour burden or extent from iUPD occurs, the status would still be iUPD. This allows delayed response following pseudo-progression to be identified.

Conclusion and learning points

- Acral lentiginous melanomas typically exhibit a different morphological, epidemiological and genetic mutational pattern of disease from that of CM.
- Responses to CTLA-4 and PD-1 immune checkpoint inhibitors have been observed in metastatic acral melanoma.
- Four radiological treatment responses ascribed to immunotherapy are:
  - a reduction in size of baseline lesions;
  - new lesions occurring at the same time as a response in other lesions;
  - an initial increase in the size of lesions followed later by a response;
  - stable and durable disease.
- Patients receiving immunotherapy should have their radiological response assessed by specific immune response criteria such as iRECIST.

References

1   Furney SJ, Turailic S, Stamp G, *et al.* Genome sequencing of mucosal melanomas reveals that they are driven by distinct mechanisms from cutaneous melanoma. *J Pathol* 2013; 230: 261–9.

2   Curtin JA, Busam K, Pinkel D, *et al.* Somatic activation of KIT in distinct subtypes of melanoma. *J Clin Oncol* 2006; 24: 4340–6.

3   Furney SJ, Turailic S, Stamp G, *et al.* The mutational burden of acral melanoma revealed by whole-genome sequencing and comparative analysis. *Pigment Cell Melanoma Res* 2014; 27: 835–8.

4   Bello DM, Chou JF, Panageas KS, *et al.* Prognosis of acral melanoma: a series of 281 patients. *Ann Surg Oncol* 2013; 20: 3618–25.

5   Shoushtari AN, Munhoz RR, Kud D, *et al.* The efficacy of anti-PD-1 agents in acral and mucosal melanoma. *Cancer* 2016; 122: 3354–62.

6   Johnson DB, Peng C, Abramson RG, *et al.* Clinical activity of ipilimumab in acral melanoma: a retrospective review. *Oncologist* 2015; 20: 648–52.

7   Brahmer JR, Tykodi SS, Chow LQ, *et al.* Safety and activity of anti-PD-L1 antibody in patients with advanced cancer. *N Engl J Med* 2012; 366: 2455–65.

8   Wolchok JD, Hoos A, O'Day S, *et al.* Guidelines for the evaluation of immune therapy activity in solid tumors: immune-related response criteria. *Clin Cancer Res* 2009; 15: 7412–20.

9   Nichino M, Tirumani SH, Ramaiya NH, *et al.* Cancer immunotherapy and immune-related response assessment: the role of radiologists in the new arena of cancer treatment. *Eur J Radiol* 2015; 84: 1259–68.

10 Di Giacomo AM, Danielli R, Guidoboni M, *et al.* Therapeutic efficacy of ipilimumab, an anti-CTLA-4 monoclonal antibody, in patients with metastatic melanoma unresponsive to prior systemic treatments: clinical and immunological evidence from three patient cases. *Cancer Immunol Immunother* 2009; 58: 1297–306.

11 Hodi FS, Hwu WJ, Kefford R, *et al.* Evaluation of immune-related response criteria and RECIST v1.1 in patients with advanced melanoma treated with pembrolizumab. *J Clin Oncol* 2016; 34: 1510–17.

12 Schreiber RD, Old LJ, Smyth MJ. Cancer immunoediting: integrating immunity's roles in cancer suppression and promotion. *Science* 2011; 331: 1565–70.

13 Chiou VL, Burotto M. Pseudoprogression and immune-related response in solid tumors. *J Clin Oncol* 2015; 33: 3541–3.

14 Seymour L, Bogaerts J, Perrone A, *et al.* iRECIST: guidelines for response criteria for use in trials testing immunotherapeutics. *Lancet Oncol* 2017; 18: e143–52.

16 Facial Nerve Palsy in a Patient with Renal Cell Carcinoma Treated with Nivolumab

Alison May Berner, Romaana Mir, Anand Sharma, Paul D. Nathan

Case history

A 64-year-old man presented with a 4 week history of haematuria. His medical history included hypertension, type 2 diabetes mellitus and ischaemic heart disease. Investigations revealed a large exophytic mass in the left kidney consistent with renal cell carcinoma (RCC). CT body staging was unremarkable. He underwent laparoscopic left nephrectomy; the final postoperative staging was pT3a left grade 2 clear cell RCC. Since this was high-risk disease, his follow-up was according to the high-risk protocol, which involved 3 monthly clinic review and 6 monthly CT imaging.

Two years into his follow-up, a solitary enlarging lung nodule was seen on the surveillance CT, which was treated with radiofrequency ablation, with confirmed response on subsequent imaging.

Subsequently he developed left arm pain. Shoulder MRI confirmed metastatic disease in the left proximal humerus. He underwent metastasectomy followed by postoperative short course radiotherapy.

During his postoperative recovery, he experienced an episode of left-sided facial weakness and was diagnosed with Bell's palsy. Symptoms resolved following a 7 day course of low-dose oral prednisolone prescribed by his GP.

He continued on watchful waiting. Four years from the diagnosis he developed multiple lobulated lung lesions, consistent with metastases, and an enlarged right adrenal gland. He was commenced on 800 mg oral pazopanib once daily and had an initial response at 3 months; however, progression developed in the known sites of disease at 6 months. In view of the disease progression, pazopanib was stopped and he started nivolumab 3 mg/kg every 2 weeks. He experienced grade 1 fatigue; random cortisol and thyroid function were within the normal range.

After cycle 5 of nivolumab he developed a second episode of left-sided facial weakness. On examination he had a left-sided facial droop with forehead sparing and weakness of left eye closure. Symptoms were consistent with left lower motor neurone facial nerve palsy. Examination of the remainder of the cranial nerves and neurological system was unremarkable. There was no ear pain or evidence of infection on otoscopy.

Head MRI showed no evidence of intracranial metastatic disease but some mild small vessel disease. A CT scan of the chest, abdomen and pelvis revealed progression at known sites of disease.

Nivolumab was stopped and following specialist neurology consultation the patient was commenced on 60 mg oral prednisolone (1 mg/kg per day), with a plan to wean by 10 mg per week. Following 4 weeks of corticosteroid treatment, he had only partial resolution of his symptoms, so his weaning regimen was modified to 5 mg per week. He was then started on cabozantinib for the progressing RCC.

At 8 weeks post-presentation his symptoms had resolved, corticosteroids were stopped and he was tolerating cabozantinib well.

What are the most likely differential diagnoses in this patient?

What tests would you perform to exclude the likely differentials?

How should neurological immune-related adverse events (irAEs) be managed?

How should refractory or worsening neurological symptoms be managed?

What are the concerns with use of corticosteroids in this patient?

What are the most likely differential diagnoses in this patient?

Differential diagnoses for left lower motor neurone facial nerve palsy in this patient include recurrent idiopathic (Bell's palsy), metastasis to the posterior fossa or parotid gland, viral infection (herpes simplex, herpes zoster, cytomegalovirus, Epstein–Barr virus and HIV) and mononeuritis multiplex resulting from diabetes mellitus or immunotherapy.

Less likely causes include Lyme disease, otitis media, cholesteatoma, trauma, multiple sclerosis and Sjögren's syndrome.

What tests would you perform to exclude the likely differentials?

MRI of the head is essential to rule out a metastatic cause and should be a priority in a patient with known history of cancer.

Bell's palsy is a diagnosis of exclusion and it may be that this man's previous presentation was in fact a mononeuritis related to his diabetes mellitus.

Although not diagnostic, HbA1c and fasting blood glucose should be checked. Serology for herpes viruses and Lyme disease should also be performed, along with HIV antibodies. Nerve conduction studies are not performed routinely as, although prognostic, they do not influence management.

Although this patient had a history of Bell's palsy, his symptoms in the second episode took much longer to resolve, implying the nerve palsy was exacerbated and/or caused by nivolumab.

How should neurological irAEs be managed?

Neurological irAEs occur in 6.1% of patients receiving anti-programmed cell death protein 1 (PD-1) therapy and in 12% with combination anti-PD-1/anti-cytotoxic T lymphocyte-associated protein 4 (CTLA-4).[1] Onset is usually rapid (median 6–13 weeks since the start of immunotherapy), but there is a wide range, and symptoms may develop many months after treatment has been discontinued.

There is a broad spectrum of presenting symptoms including mononeuritis multiplex, ascending polyneuropathy (Guillain–Barré), demyelinating disease and myasthenia gravis. Isolated nerve palsy may be the first presentation of a progressive neurological toxicity.

Immunotherapy should be withheld until the patient has been stabilized and other causative factors excluded. Careful consideration should be taken before restarting immunotherapy. For low-grade toxicity (grade 1) oral prednisolone (1 mg/kg per day) should be prescribed with urgent onward referral to neurology.[1,2] In the case of isolated facial nerve palsy, antivirals are not recommended in the absence of clinical or serological evidence of viral infection.

How should refractory or worsening neurological symptoms be managed?

Patients with higher-grade toxicity (grade ≥2) and those with progressive neurology or low-grade symptoms refractory to oral corticosteroids should be escalated to intravenous methylprednisolone (1–2 mg/kg per day). Neurology referral is essential. Intravenous immunoglobulin may be considered in patients with severe symptoms (e.g. myasthenia gravis or Guillain–Barré) but is unlikely to be used in isolated mononeuritis that is non-progressive.[3,4] Patients with high-grade neurological toxicity are best managed in a neurological specialist unit, as regular monitoring of neurology and forced vital capacity is essential.

What are the concerns with use of corticosteroids in this patient?

High-dose, prolonged steroid treatment is likely to affect diabetic control and may necessitate up-titration of oral glucose-lowering medications and specialist referral to endocrinology. In our experience, many patients require the addition of insulin to their diabetic regimen; insulin may often be stopped following completion of the corticosteroid course.

Conclusion and learning points

- The incidence of neurological irAEs is 6% for single-agent anti-PD-1 and 12% for combination anti-PD-1/anti-CTLA-4.

- The incidence of neurological irAEs may be increased in those with a previous neurological condition.

- In lower motor neurone facial nerve palsy, early head MRI is essential to exclude metastatic disease as a cause of symptoms.

- Initial treatment for immunotherapy-related mononeuritis is oral prednisolone (1 mg/kg per day).

- Early isolated neuropathies may be an early sign prior to the emergence of progressive neurological irAEs, which may require high-dose intravenous corticosteroids and in severe cases intravenous immunoglobulin.

References

1 Haanen JBAG, Carbonnel F, Robert C, *et al*. Management of toxicities from immunotherapy: ESMO clinical practice guidelines for diagnosis, treatment and follow-up. *Ann Oncol* 2017; 28 (suppl 4): iv119–42.

2 Puzanov I, Diab A, Abdallah K, *et al*. Managing toxicities associated with immune checkpoint inhibitors: consensus recommendations from the Society for Immunotherapy of Cancer (SITC) Toxicity Management Working Group. *J Immunother Cancer* 2017; 5: 95.

3 Kelly Wu W, Broman KK, Brownie ER, Kauffmann RM. Ipilimumab-induced Guillain–Barré syndrome presenting as dysautonomia: an unusual presentation of a rare complication of immunotherapy. *J Immunother* 2017; 40: 196–9.

4 Patel RJ, Liu MA, Amaraneni A, Sindhu SK. Rare side effect of adjuvant ipilimumab after surgical resection of melanoma: Guillain–Barré syndrome. *BMJ Case Study Rep* 2017; 2017. pii: bcr-2017–221318.

Further reading

- Astaras C, de Micheli R, Moura B, *et al*. Neurological adverse events associated with immune checkpoint inhibitors: diagnosis and management. *Curr Neurol Neurosci* 2018; 18: 3.

17 Acute Kidney Injury in a Patient on Combination Immunotherapy for Metastatic Melanoma

Romaana Mir, Alison May Berner, Heather M. Shaw, Paul D. Nathan

Case history

A 76-year-old man presented with a left submandibular mass. His medical history included type 2 diabetes mellitus and pulmonary embolism.

Ultrasound of the left neck and fine needle aspiration cytology demonstrated an enlarged lymph node containing malignant melanoma. Total skin examination was unremarkable, as was the staging CT of the body and MRI of the head and neck. He underwent excision of the lymph node together with radical left neck dissection, which confirmed no further spread of the cancer. The melanoma was *BRAF* and *NRAS* wild-type.

As he was at high risk of cancer relapse the specialist melanoma multidisciplinary team recommended surveillance 6 monthly CT body imaging alongside MRI head and neck.

While on surveillance, he developed multiple small-volume lung metastases. He was asymptomatic. He received combination ipilimumab (3 mg/kg) and nivolumab (1 mg/kg) immunotherapy 3 weekly and underwent repeat imaging after cycle 4, which demonstrated a partial response to treatment.

He continued with immunotherapy with maintenance nivolumab 3 mg/kg every 2 weeks. After two cycles his renal function deteriorated from baseline creatinine 94 µmol/l to 175 µmol/l. He was well and had no radiological evidence of disease progression, dehydration or infection. He had not been started on new medication. Maintenance nivolumab was stopped.

He was commenced on 70 mg oral prednisolone (1 mg/kg per day) but his renal function deteriorated further with a creatinine rise to 212 µmol/l. As his renal function was refractory to oral corticosteroids, he was commenced on oral mycophenolate mofetil 1 g twice daily, together with the pre-existing dose of oral prednisolone.

His creatinine level improved steadily over a 4 week period to 188 µmol/l and plateaued at 148–135 µmol/l. The corticosteroid dose was weaned by 10 mg per week and he continues with 10 mg oral prednisolone and mycophenolate mofetil while awaiting interval imaging.

What is the initial work-up for acute kidney injury (AKI)?

What is the optimal management of immunotherapy-induced AKI?

What factors are important when considering the need for renal replacement therapy?

What is the evidence for the effect of combination immunosuppression on metastatic melanoma?

What is the initial work-up for AKI?

Acute management of AKI includes evaluation of fluid status, acid-base balance and imaging to diagnose urinary obstruction or disease progression. Life-threatening uraemia and hyperkalaemia should be excluded. Urine dipstick should be performed along with urine microscopy for casts, crystals and culture. Vasculitic and autoimmune profile should be requested to exclude an intrinsic renal cause.

What is the optimal management of immunotherapy-induced AKI?

Immunotherapy rarely causes AKI. The incidence of AKI is 4.9% with combination anti-programmed cell death protein 1 (PD-1) and anti-cytotoxic T lymphocyte-associated protein 4 (CTLA-4) therapy, and 0.4% and 1.4% with anti-CTLA-4 and anti-PD-1 single agents, respectively.[1-3]

Clinical presentation is varied. In this case, the patient was asymptomatic with deteriorating renal function noted on a standard of care blood test prior to the nivolumab. Other potential presentations include haematuria, escalating uncontrolled hypertension, sub-nephrotic proteinuria or microscopic pyuria.[4] Microscopically, immunotherapy-induced AKI resembles acute interstitial nephritis, with case series consistently demonstrating the presence of activated clusters of differentiation (CD)4+ T lymphocytes in the renal parenchyma.[4]

Immunotherapy should be discontinued in all cases. Oral corticosteroids (prednisolone 0.5–1 mg/kg per day) are recommended and should be weaned to nil once renal function has improved. In the main, an 8 week course of weaning corticosteroids should be sufficient to resolve the AKI.[4,5]

Management of progressive or relapsing renal function should include involvement of tertiary services with a low threshold for renal biopsy, as biopsy will exclude primary renal pathology and guide further management.

In this case, oral mycophenolate mofetil was effective in recapturing renal function improvement refractory to high-dose corticosteroids. Mycophenolate mofetil is a pro-drug of mycophenolic acid, which in turn directly inhibits activated T and B lymphocytes.[6] Current indications for mycophenolate mofetil include prophylaxis of acute transplant rejection and management of corticosteroid and infliximab refractory colitis. Although the use of mycophenolate mofetil in the management of immunotherapy-induced AKI is a non-standard approach, mycophenolate mofetil was effective in achieving and sustaining improvement in renal function in this case.

What factors are important when considering the need for renal replacement therapy?

Haemodialysis is indicated in cases of refractory hyperkalaemia, uraemia and fluid overload. Haemodialysis should be considered carefully in patients with established metastatic malignancy, and a multidisciplinary approach should be taken when starting such renal replacement therapy.

Restaging CT chest, abdomen and pelvis should be performed to establish response, as some patients will have disease stability and achieve a durable response to immunotherapy. Renal replacement therapy may be only a short-term holding measure while immunosuppression takes effect;[5] however, the morbidity of long-term renal replacement therapy should be discussed with all patients.

What is the evidence for the effect of combination immunosuppression on metastatic melanoma?

Immunosuppression forms the backbone of treatment for immune-related adverse events (irAEs). The long-term effects of immunosuppression on the patient and melanoma are debated. Although there are concerns that systemic immunosuppression may counteract the effects of immunotherapy on the cancer, a retrospective review of 298 patients with metastatic melanoma indicated no significant effect on time to treatment failure or overall survival in those who received high-dose corticosteroids.[7]

Prolonged courses of corticosteroids may cause significant morbidity including corticosteroid-induced diabetes, suppression of the hypothalamic–pituitary–adrenal axis, weight gain, insomnia and fatigue. A multidisciplinary approach is advised to monitor and manage these treatment-induced side effects.

Conclusion and learning points

- The incidence of renal irAEs with combination immunotherapy is 4.9%.
- Renal function should be checked prior to each cycle of immunotherapy.
- Renal irAEs may be asymptomatic, but presentation may be varied and include haematuria, escalating uncontrolled hypertension, sub-nephrotic proteinuria or microscopic pyuria.
- All patients on immunotherapy presenting with AKI require full assessment to exclude non-immunotherapy-related causes. Nephrology referral and renal biopsy are indicated in cases of diagnostic uncertainty.
- Renal irAEs respond well to 0.5–1 mg/kg oral prednisolone. The corticosteroid dose should be weaned over 8 weeks.
- Corticosteroid refractory renal irAEs warrant urgent referral to a tertiary renal unit, with consideration given to commencing steroid-sparing immunosuppressants and renal replacement therapy.

References

1   Robert C, Schachter J, Long GV, *et al.* Pembrolizumab versus ipilimumab in advanced melanoma. *N Engl J Med* 2015; 372: 2521–32.

2   Larkin J, Chiarion-Sileni V, González R, *et al.* Combined nivolumab and ipilimumab or monotherapy in untreated melanoma. *N Engl J Med* 2015; 373: 23–34.

3   Hodi FS, Chesney J, Pavlick AC, *et al.* Combined nivolumab and ipilimumab versus ipilimumab alone in patients with advanced melanoma: 2-year overall survival outcomes in a multicentre, randomised, controlled, phase 2 trial. *Lancet Oncol* 2016; 17: 1558–68.

4   Cortazar FB, Marrone KA, Troxell ML, *et al.* Clinicopathological features of acute kidney injury associated with immune checkpoint inhibitors. *Kidney Int* 2016; 90: 638–47.

5   Haanen JBAG, Carbonnel F, Robert C, *et al.* Management of toxicities from immunotherapy: ESMO clinical practice guidelines for diagnosis, treatment and follow-up. *Ann Oncol* 2017; 28 (suppl 4): iv119–42.

6   Allison AC, Eugui EM. Mycophenolate mofetil and its mechanism of action. *Immunopharmacology* 2000; 47: 85–118.

7   Horvat TZ, Adel NG, Dang TO, *et al.* Immune-related adverse events, need for systemic immunosuppression, and effects on survival and time to treatment failure in patients with melanoma treated with ipilimumab at Memorial Sloan Kettering Cancer Center. *J Clin Oncol* 2015; 33: 3193–8.

Further reading

•   Murakami N, Motwani S, Riella LV. Renal complications of immune checkpoint blockade. *Curr Probl Cancer* 2017; 41: 100–10.

18 Immune Pneumonitis after Immunotherapy for Metastatic Melanoma

Dan R. Muller, Marcus Remer, Sunnya Zarif, Matthew Wheater, Christian Ottensmeier

Case history

A 69-year-old man with a history of stage IV melanoma presented with a 3 week history of dyspnoea. He had been diagnosed with a stage III melanoma, *BRAF* wild-type, 4 years previously and had undergone a radical resection with lymph node dissection, followed by surveillance. After 3 years he presented with a gastrointestinal bleed, leading to the diagnosis of small bowel recurrence. He underwent palliative bowel surgery; however, radiological assessment confirmed residual nodal and likely bowel disease. He was commenced on dual immunotherapy with ipilimumab and nivolumab. He completed four cycles of combination immunotherapy followed by maintenance anti-programmed cell death protein 1 (PD-1) monotherapy. Restaging contrast CT showed a good response with near complete resolution of disease. Immunotherapy was discontinued because of immune-related toxicity with colitis and hypophysitis.

Five months after completion of immunotherapy, the patient was hospitalized with breathlessness. Chest X-ray showed bilateral patchy consolidation in the mid- and lower zones. CT chest demonstrated confluent ground glass change and diffuse pan-lobar patchy consolidation with a peribronchial distribution. The differential diagnosis included atypical infection, immunotherapy-induced pneumonitis and tumour-related infiltrative lymphangiosis. The patient received intravenous antibiotics and oxygen therapy but deteriorated, developing life-threatening type 1 respiratory failure requiring invasive ventilation on the intensive care ward. He was started on intravenous high-dose co-trimoxazole for *Pneumocystis jirovecii* pneumonia based on the CT changes and history of steroid use for previous immune-mediated toxicity. A diagnosis of immunotherapy-induced pneumonitis was considered and he was commenced on intravenous steroids, albeit at a reduced dose because of reluctance from the intensive care physicians (0.7 mg/kg per day methylprednisolone equivalent).

The patient's respiratory function improved and he was extubated, unfortunately prior to invasive sputum sampling: although routine sputum returned negative for atypical organisms and respiratory viruses, expectorated sputum alone was insufficient to exclude a diagnosis of *P. jirovecii* pneumonia.

Despite his improving breathlessness, diagnostic bronchoscopy was performed to ascertain the underlying aetiology. Histology showed only minor reactive changes with no evidence of pneumonitis and no malignant cells. Microbiology was negative for all organisms tested, including *Legionella*, *Mycoplasma* and *P. jirovecii* pneumonia. He was switched to alternative oral antibiotics and a reducing course of oral steroids. His breathing improved and he no longer required oxygen. At last review in early 2018, he remained fully recovered and in remission from his melanoma.

What is the evidence base for the use of dual immunotherapy in this patient?

What is the survival benefit of using maintenance therapy after dual immunotherapy?

What is the likelihood of developing life-threatening respiratory complications after dual immunotherapy?

Why was there such diagnostic uncertainty in treating this patient's respiratory illness?

What is the evidence base for the use of dual immunotherapy in this patient?

Dual immunotherapy with ipilimumab (anti-cytotoxic T lymphocyte-associated protein 4 [CTLA-4] monoclonal antibody) plus nivolumab (anti-PD-1 monoclonal antibody) has become the gold standard of treatment for patients with stage IV melanoma. Several landmark phase III clinical trials have demonstrated a significant survival benefit with dual immunotherapy over conventional chemotherapy[1,2] and anti-CTLA-4 monotherapy.[3,4] The incidence of serious or life-threatening immune-related adverse events (irAEs) increases, however, with combination therapy.

CheckMate 067 (2015–2017)

This US-based, global, phase III, randomized, double-blind trial was conducted to evaluate the safety and efficacy of nivolumab alone, nivolumab plus ipilimumab, or ipilimumab alone.[3,4] The trial recruited 945 previously treated patients with unresectable stage III or IV melanoma and allocated treatment arms in a 1:1:1 ratio. Combination ipilimumab/nivolumab prolonged median progression-free survival (PFS) to 11.5 months, compared with 2.9 months with ipilimumab alone (HR 0.42; 99.5% CI 0.31, 0.57; $p<0.001$). Nivolumab alone prolonged PFS to 6.9 months, compared with 2.9 months with ipilimumab alone (HR 0.57; 99.5% CI 0.43, 0.76; $p<0.001$). Grade 3 or 4 irAEs occurred in 55.0% of patients treated with ipilimumab plus nivolumab, and in 27.3% and 16.3% in the ipilimumab and nivolumab groups, respectively. At a minimum follow-up of 36 months, the median overall survival (OS) had not been reached in the combination group, median OS was 37.6 months in the nivolumab group and 19.9 months in the ipilimumab group: HR for death with ipilimumab/nivolumab vs ipilimumab alone, 0.55 ($p<0.001$); HR for death with nivolumab vs ipilimumab, 0.65 ($p<0.001$). The 3 year OS rate was 58% in the combination group, 52% in the nivolumab group and 34% in the ipilimumab group. Grade 3 or 4 irAEs remained comparable and occurred in 59% of patients receiving combination treatment, 21% in the nivolumab group and 28% in the ipilimumab group.

CA209–004 trial

This US-based, phase I dose-escalation study investigated the clinical activity of concurrent therapy with nivolumab and ipilimumab in patients with previously treated or untreated advanced melanoma.[5] Concurrent cohorts of patients received escalating doses of 3 weekly ipilimumab/

nivolumab for four doses, followed by 3 weekly nivolumab for four doses, followed by maintenance 12 weekly ipilimumab/nivolumab for eight doses ($n=53$). An expansion cohort received 3
weekly ipilimumab/nivolumab for four doses, followed by maintenance 12 weekly nivolumab for
eight doses ($n=41$). Three year OS data were published in 2018. At a minimum follow-up of 30
months, the 3 year OS rate was 69% and the median OS had not been reached for the concurrent
treatment cohorts. The objective response rate was 43%, with a median duration of response of
22.3 months. The incidence of treatment-related grades 3 and 4 toxicity was 59%.

What is the survival benefit of using maintenance therapy after dual immunotherapy?

The current practice of using maintenance anti-PD-1 therapy after completion of initial combination
immunotherapy follows the protocol used in CheckMate 067.[3,4] After combination immunotherapy,
48 patients enrolled in the CheckMate 067 study went on to receive subsequent immunotherapy,
32 with an anti-PD-1 agent.[4] The number of doses of nivolumab given after completion of four
cycles of dual immunotherapy ranged from 0 to 90 (maximum duration of maintenance treatment approximately 42 months). The rationale behind this is to increase exposure to immunotherapy while reducing the risk of toxicity by using anti-PD-1 medication, which has a lower irAE
profile[3,4] and has been shown to increase survival in ipilimumab refractory disease.[6]

What is the likelihood of developing life–threatening respiratory complications after dual immunotherapy?

Respiratory complications, despite not being the most common, are a well-recognized immunotherapy toxicity, pneumonitis being the most significant of these. Immune-mediated pneumonitis
is caused by an interstitial, granulomatous, fibrosing inflammation of the lung, especially of the
bronchioles and alveoli.[7] It commonly presents with dyspnoea and/or dry cough. Radiographic
features are normally non-specific but include ground glass changes, air-space opacification and
reticulonodular shadowing. These may occur in a variety of patterns depending on the underlying
aetiology of the pneumonitis but are frequently bilateral and diffuse in nature.[8]

Immune-related pneumonitis is potentially fatal and was the cause of three deaths in early trials
of PD-1 inhibitors.[9] Pneumonitis is most commonly seen in combination immunotherapy. When
using single-agent immunotherapy, pneumonitis is more prevalent after anti-PD-1 than after anti-
CTLA-4 treatment.[10] In a pooled analysis investigating the irAEs of PD-1 inhibitors, pneumonitis
was the most common event leading to discontinuation of therapy.[11] Pneumonitis may occur at
any time; however, it appears to occur later compared with irAEs in other organ systems and, as
in our case, may occur months after treatment is initiated.[12]

Pooled analysis of phase II and III trials looking at the safety of dual immunotherapy in advanced melanoma found that of the 407 patients included, 10 (2.5%) developed immune-mediated
pneumonitis, four (1%) of which were grade 3 or 4.[13] In the CheckMate 067 study, at the time of
the first report in 2015, 32 of the 313 (10.2%) patients in the combination treatment cohort had
developed pneumonitis, with grades 3–4 pneumonitis occurring in two patients (0.6%).[3] At a
minimum follow-up of 30 months, 36 patients (12%) had developed pneumonitis of any grade,
and three patients (1%) had developed grades 3–4 toxicity.[4]

Why was there such diagnostic uncertainty in treating this patient's respiratory illness?

The differential diagnosis of dyspnoea and diffuse pulmonary changes in this patient was
complex, given the previous treatment with immune checkpoint inhibitors, immune toxicity leading to prolonged steroid use and the underlying history of malignancy. Prolonged glucocorticoid

administration may lead to immunosuppression by inhibition of cytokine gene expression and the decreased release of interleukins, interferons and tumour necrosis factor.[14] Such patients are susceptible to infection by a varying range of organisms (bacterial, viral, fungal) compared with immune-competent individuals.[15]

Rapid diagnosis and initiation of appropriate therapy are the basis of successful management of infection in the immunocompromised patient. It is important to be aggressive in pursuing a specific microbiological diagnosis, to enable prompt initiation of therapy while avoiding the use of overly-broad antimicrobial therapy. A specific diagnosis avoids the potential toxicities of broad-spectrum antimicrobial therapies, most notably nephrotoxicity and *Clostridium difficile* colitis, and the potential pitfalls from drug interactions.[16] This also confirms the underlying diagnosis as an infective, rather than a non-infective cause, such as drug-induced immune-mediated pneumonitis.

Invasive procedures are frequently required to obtain tissue or sputum in order to make a specific diagnosis. Decisions regarding invasive procedures are best made early in the management course, since patients may become too ill or develop contraindications (e.g. coagulopathy, hypoxaemia) that prevent the ability to perform procedures later on.[17,18]

While it is desirable to seek a single unifying diagnosis for a patient's respiratory compromise, it is always possible for multiple aetiologies to coexist.[16] An infective cause of infiltrative lung disease may be superimposed on a non-infective cause, with the underlying pathology increasing the susceptibility to an infective organism.

Conclusion and learning points

- Dual immunotherapy conveys a survival benefit over both single-agent immunotherapy and previous conventional therapies for metastatic melanoma.

- The risk of developing severe immune-related toxicity is increased with combination immunotherapy compared with monotherapy (59% vs 21–28%).

- Respiratory complications are not uncommon with combination immunotherapy (2.5–12%) and are potentially fatal.

- Patients on long-term steroid medication are at increased risk of developing atypical infections that may complicate the differential diagnosis of respiratory compromise following immunotherapy.

- Invasive investigation with bronchoscopy (tissue sampling, lavage for microscopy, virology) is beneficial in obtaining a diagnosis to allow for definitive management to be instigated promptly.

- A single unifying cause of the underlying disease may not be found and the aetiology of pulmonary compromise in the immunocompromised patient may be multifactorial (immune-mediated pneumonitis with super-added atypical infection).

References

1 Robert C, Thomas L, Bondarenko I, *et al*. Ipilimumab plus dacarbazine for previously untreated metastatic melanoma. *N Engl J Med* 2011; 364: 2517–26.

2 Hodi FS, O'Day SJ, McDermott DF, *et al*. Improved survival with ipilimumab in patients with metastatic melanoma. *N Engl J Med* 2010; 363: 711–23.

3   Larkin J, Hodi FS, Wolchok JD. Combined nivolumab and ipilimumab or monotherapy in untreated melanoma. *N Engl J Med* 2015; 373: 1270–1.

4   Wolchok J, Chiarion-Sileni V, González R, *et al.* Overall survival with combined nivolumab and ipilimumab in advanced melanoma. *N Engl J Med* 2017; 377: 1345–56.

5   Callahan MK, Kluger H, Postow MA, *et al.* Nivolumab plus ipilimumab in patients with advanced melanoma: updated survival, response, and safety data in a phase I dose-escalation study. *J Clin Oncol* 2018; 36: 391–8.

6   Hamid O, Puzanov I, Dummer R, *et al.* Final analysis of a randomised trial comparing pembrolizumab versus investigator-choice chemotherapy for ipilimumab-refractory advanced melanoma. *Eur J Cancer* 2017; 86: 37–45.

7   O'Toole M. Pneumonitis. *Mosby's medical dictionary.* 8th ed. Maryland Heights, MO: Elsevier, 2009; 1470.

8   Weerakkody Y (2018). *Hypersensitivity pneumonitis.* Available from: https://radiopaedia.org/articles/hypersensitivity-pneumonitis (accessed 21 June 2018).

9   Topalian SL, Hodi FS, Brahmer JR, *et al.* Safety, activity, and immune correlates of anti-PD-1 antibody in cancer. *N Engl J Med* 2012; 366: 2443–54.

10   Robert C, Schachter J, Long GV, *et al.* Pembrolizumab versus ipilimumab in advanced melanoma. *N Engl J Med* 2015; 372: 2521–32.

11   Eigentler TK, Hassel JC, Berking C, *et al.* Diagnosis, monitoring and management of immune-related adverse drug reactions of anti-PD-1 antibody therapy. *Cancer Treat Rev* 2016; 45: 7–18.

12   Haanen JBAG, Carbonnel F, Robert C, *et al.* Management of toxicities from immunotherapy: ESMO clinical practice guidelines for diagnosis, treatment and follow-up. *Ann Oncol* 2017; 28: 119–42.

13   Schadendorf D, Wolchok J, Hodi FS, *et al.* Efficacy and safety outcomes in patients with advanced melanoma who discontinued treatment with nivolumab and ipilimumab because of adverse events: a pooled analysis of randomized phase II and III trials. *J Clin Oncol* 2017; 35: 3807–14.

14   Meier CA. Mechanisms of immunosuppression by glucocorticoids. *Eur J Endocrinol* 1996; 134: 50.

15   Arriola E, Wheater M, Krishnan R, *et al.* Immunosuppression for ipilimumab-related toxicity can cause *Pneumocystis* pneumonia but spare antitumor immune control. *OncoImmunol* 2015; 4: e1040218.

16   Fishman JA (2017). *Approach to the immunocompromised patient with fever and pulmonary infiltrates.* Available from: www.uptodate.com/contents/approach-to-the-immunocompromised-patient-with-fever-and-pulmonary-infiltrates (accessed 22 February 2018).

17   Shannon VR, Andersson BS, Lei X, *et al.* Utility of early versus late fiberoptic bronchoscopy in the evaluation of new pulmonary infiltrates following hematopoietic stem cell transplantation. *Bone Marrow Transplant* 2010; 45: 647–55.

18   Chellapandian D, Lehrnbecher T, Phillips B, *et al.* Bronchoalveolar lavage and lung biopsy in patients with cancer and hematopoietic stem-cell transplantation recipients: a systematic review and meta-analysis. *J Clin Oncol* 2015; 33: 501–9.

Further reading

- Blansfield JA, Beck KE, Tran K, *et al.* Cytotoxic T-lymphocyte-associated antigen-4 blockage may induce autoimmune hypophysitis in patients with metastatic melanoma and renal cancer. *J Immunother* 2005; 28: 593–8.

- Brahmer JR, Lacchetti C, Schneider BJ, *et al.* Management of immune-related adverse events in patients treated with immune checkpoint inhibitor therapy: American Society of Clinical Oncology clinical practice guideline. *J Clin Oncol* 2018; 36: 1714–68.

- Nishino M, Ramaiya N, Awad M, *et al.* PD-1 inhibitor-related pneumonitis in advanced cancer patients: radiographic patterns and clinical course. *Clin Cancer Res* 2016; 22: 6051–60.

19 A Patient with Ureteric Transitional Cell Carcinoma on Anti-PD-1 Antibody Complicated by Sarcoidosis

Pavlina Spiliopoulou, Rob J. Jones

Case history

A 79-year-old man was found to have thickening of the right ureter during staging investigations for a Dukes' A rectal adenocarcinoma. Ureteroscopy revealed a grade 3 transitional cell carcinoma of the distal right ureter as well as a suspicious lung nodule. The primary ureteric tumour was deemed inoperable and the patient was referred to oncology for consideration of systemic treatment. His medical history consisted of chronic obstructive pulmonary disease, osteoarthritis and hypertension. He had a right-sided ureteric stent *in situ* with established right kidney cortical atrophy and borderline creatinine clearance.

He was not considered suitable for cisplatin-based chemotherapy (the current standard of care for advanced urothelial cancer); he therefore received six cycles of carboplatin/ gemcitabine, with partial response. Fifteen months later he developed progressive metastasis in the upper lobe of the right lung. He entered an early phase clinical trial with the anti-programmed cell death protein 1 (PD-1) antibody nivolumab.

Early in the treatment he developed grade 1 pruritus, managed with topical steroids, and a grade 3 asymptomatic amylase rise that subsequently resolved without intervention. His disease remained stable for 10 months, when a CT scan revealed evolving mediastinal and abdominal lymphadenopathy. In the absence of new clinical findings and/or unacceptable toxicity, treatment was continued based on the possibility that the new lymphadenopathy could be attributed to pseudo-progression. At the same time he complained of small joint arthralgia in both hands, which was adequately managed with analgesia.

Over the next 18 months the size of mediastinal and abdominal lymphadenopathy fluctuated by a few millimetres, while the primary tumour remained stable throughout; the anti-PD-1 antibody was continued. Twenty-eight months after starting treatment the patient presented with an eruption of a pruritic, scaly rash on his arms and legs with purple plaques on his back (Figure 19.1). A skin biopsy was obtained but, before the results were available, he was admitted with symptomatic hypercalcaemia (corrected calcium 3 mmol/l [normal range 2.20–2.60 mmol/l]). The biopsy results showed granulomatous dermatitis in the superficial dermis with negative stains for mycobacteria and negative stains for fungal infection. The changes were pathognomonic of cutaneous sarcoidosis. CT imaging of the chest showed reticulonodular lung parenchymal changes consistent with interstitial lung disease (Figure 19.2).

The combination of interstitial lung changes, cutaneous sarcoidosis and hypercalcaemia established the diagnosis of systemic sarcoidosis. All changes resolved with the withdrawal of nivolumab; the patient's cancer remained stable when last seen 6 months after discontinuation of immunotherapy.

On what basis was the patient deemed unsuitable for first line cisplatin-based chemotherapy, and what is the evidence behind the use of platinum/gemcitabine in urothelial cancer?

What is the role of nivolumab and other immunotherapeutic agents in the second line treatment of urothelial cancer?

What are the commonest toxicities associated with anti-PD-1 antibodies, and what is the mainstay of their treatment?

How common is sarcoidosis with anti-PD-1 treatment, and how does it present?

A   B

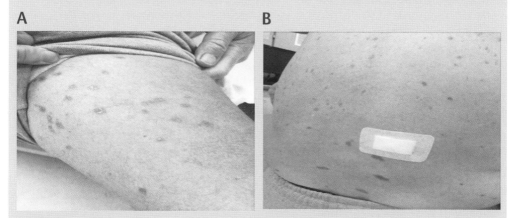

Figure 19.1 (A) Pruritic, scaly rash on the patient's legs and (B) purple plaques on his back.

A   B

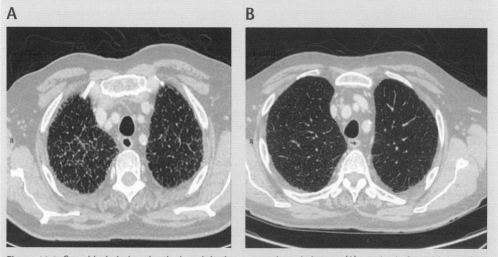

Figure 19.2 Sarcoidosis-induced reticulonodular lung parenchymal changes (A), resolved after withdrawal of immunotherapy (B).

On what basis was the patient deemed unsuitable for first line cisplatin–based chemotherapy, and what is the evidence behind the use of platinum/gemcitabine in urothelial cancer?

Urothelial cancer (cancer of the bladder, ureter or renal pelvis) is a disease that predominantly affects the elderly population, who often present with comorbidity. In addition, the nature of urothelial cancer means that renal impairment is particularly common at presentation. Impaired performance status or organ function (kidney, heart, hearing) is often associated with advanced age and may be exacerbated by cisplatin toxicity, making many patients unsuitable to receive this drug. In order to standardize criteria for selection of patients who are fit enough to receive cisplatin chemotherapy, oncologists have compiled a list of features that render a patient at high risk of being harmed by cisplatin-based chemotherapy. These are: Eastern Cooperative Oncology Group performance status ≤2, creatinine clearance <60 ml/s per m², grade ≤2 hearing loss, grade ≤2 peripheral neuropathy, and New York Heart Association class III heart failure.[1] These features are routinely used in clinical practice to aid decision making in first line treatment of advanced urothelial cancer; around 50% of patients are deemed unsuitable for cisplatin but still suitable for treatment.

The methotrexate, vinblastine, doxorubicin and cisplatin (MVAC) regimen was the first cisplatin-containing regimen to confer a survival advantage compared with cisplatin monotherapy, with response rates of 39% vs 12% ($p<0.0001$) and median overall survival (OS) of 12.5 months vs 8.2 months.[2,3] Compared with MVAC, the combination of gemcitabine and cisplatin has similar efficacy with regard to OS (HR 1.09; 95% CI 0.88, 1.34; $p=0.66$) but has less serious toxicity.[4] Gemcitabine/cisplatin is therefore now widely used in suitable patients. For patients who are unsuitable for cisplatin-based chemotherapy, gemcitabine/carboplatin is an alternative option.[4,5]

What is the role of nivolumab and other immunotherapeutic agents in the second line treatment of urothelial cancer?

Nivolumab is an anti-PD-1 antibody that has been tested and approved for the treatment of several cancers including urothelial carcinoma that has progressed after previous platinum-based chemotherapy. Its efficacy has been assessed in two large, early phase clinical trials, with objective responses varying between 19.6% and 24.4%, regardless of programmed death-ligand 1 (PD-L1) expression. Long-term survival data are not yet available from these non-randomized studies.[6,7] Inhibition of the PD-1/PD-L1 axis has raised a lot of interest in the second line treatment of urothelial carcinoma, and an additional four antibodies have recently been approved by the US Food and Drug Administration (pembrolizumab, atezolizumab, avelumab and durvalumab). Pembrolizumab, atezolizumab and nivolumab are approved in Europe. Pembrolizumab is the only antibody with level 1 evidence of superiority over second line chemotherapy in this setting. In a randomized phase III trial the median OS was 10.3 months vs 7.4 months (HR for death, 0.73; 95% CI 0.59, 0.91; $p=0.002$).[8]

Atezolizumab (a PD-L1 targeted antibody) has a favourable safety profile when compared with chemotherapy but has failed to demonstrate survival gain compared with chemotherapy in the PD-L1-expressing population. In the Study of Atezolizumab Compared with Chemotherapy in Participants with Locally Advanced or Metastatic Urothelial Bladder Cancer (IMvigor211), patients with high PD-L1 expression on tumour-infiltrating immune cells had a median OS of 11.1 months with atezolizumab and 10.6 months with chemotherapy (stratified HR 0.87; 95% CI 0.63, 1.21; $p=0.41$). In an exploratory analysis, however, of the intention-to-treat population (regardless of PD-L1 expression) median OS was 8.6 vs 8.0 months (HR 0.85; 95% CI 0.73, 0.99; $p=0.04$).[9]

In early phase trials, the response rates with avelumab and durvalumab were 17% and 17.8%, respectively;[10,11] however, there is a lack of randomized mature data on these compounds in the second line context for urothelial cancer.

What are the commonest toxicities associated with anti–PD-1 antibodies, and what is the mainstay of their treatment?

Immune checkpoint inhibitors (ICPIs) have revolutionized the therapeutic landscape of multiple tumour types, offering durable responses and enabling long-term survival for some patients. Despite the evolving experience in the management of their toxicity, however, immune-related adverse events (irAEs) limit their usefulness and preclude some patients from being eligible for treatment. Blocking the PD-1/PD-L1 axis may cause toxicities similar to those seen with cytotoxic T lymphocyte-associated protein 4 (CTLA-4) inhibitors such as ipilimumab, but their frequency and severity may be more favourable compared with treatment with single-agent anti-CTLA-4 or a combination of anti-PD-1/anti-CTLA-4. Commonest toxicities are cutaneous (rash/pruritus/vitiligo), diarrhoea/colitis, hepatitis, endocrinopathies (hyper/hypothyroidism, adrenal insufficiency, hypophysitis), pneumonitis, infusion reactions and arthralgia. Rarer forms of immune-mediated phenomena include nephritis, uveitis, cardiomyopathies, encephalitis and thrombocytopenia.[12]

The mainstay of treatment of irAEs is the use of corticosteroids, but other immunomodulatory agents such as infliximab and mycophenolate mofetil have specific indications following steroid failure, for example in severe colitis or hepatitis. irAEs may occur at any point after initiation of treatment, including the months after discontinuation, so heightened awareness of these issues and an understanding of the importance of prompt investigation and treatment are vital for oncologists, primary care physicians and acute medicine specialists. Physicians also need to be aware of the immunosuppressive effects of steroids and other immunomodulatory drugs and the associated risk of opportunistic infections. The theoretical risk of attenuating efficacy with the use of steroids and other immunosuppressive drugs has not been proven to have a negative effect on patients' survival outcomes.[13]

How common is sarcoidosis with anti–PD-1 treatment, and how does it present?

The incidence of sarcoidosis secondary to ICPI treatment is low, albeit not accurately documented as it is only reported anecdotally in case study series. Most of the cases reported in the literature are associated with anti-CTLA-4 blockade in melanoma patients, but there are emerging data that PD-1 inhibition may also activate the non-caseating granulomatous inflammation that characterises systemic sarcoidosis. The case described here perhaps represents the first documented in a patient with urothelial cancer and, compared with other published case studies, it is a relatively late presentation.

Sarcoidosis is an inflammatory process of unknown aetiology that manifests with the formation of non-caseating granulomas, predominantly in the lungs and intrathoracic lymph nodes. It may cause systemic symptoms (fever, anorexia), polyarthralgia, and skin manifestations such as erythema nodosum, panniculitis, lupus pernio and maculopapular plaques. Both B and T lymphocytes are implicated in the pathogenesis of sarcoidosis, which may justify the role of the PD-1/PD-L1 axis in its pathogenesis, given that PD-L1 is expressed on activated B and T immune cells.

Hypercalcaemia, as observed in our case study, may be seen in up to 13% of patients with sarcoidosis and relates to the secretion of 1,25-dihydroxycholecalciferol by the non-caseating granulomas. Steroids are the mainstay of therapy, but other immunosuppressive drugs such as methotrexate, infliximab, chloroquine, azathioprine or ciclosporin may be used if steroids fail to control the disease.

Conclusion and learning points

- Systemic therapy for advanced urothelial cancer had developed little until recently, with platinum-based combination chemotherapy being the mainstay of treatment.
- PD-1/PD-L1 targeted antibody treatments clearly benefit some patients with advanced urothelial cancer, where the prolonged duration of response translates into a significant survival benefit.
- ICPI treatment frequently results in irAEs such as colitis, pneumonitis and endocrinopathies, but rarer syndromes such as systemic sarcoidosis may occur and sometimes mimic the effects of the underlying cancer.
- irAEs may occur at any point after initiation of immunotherapy and should therefore always be considered, particularly when a patient presents with symptoms and signs that are otherwise difficult to explain.
- New lymphadenopathy while on immunotherapy may merit further investigation.

References

1 Galsky MD, Hahn NM, Rosenberg J, *et al.* A consensus definition of patients with metastatic urothelial carcinoma who are unfit for cisplatin-based chemotherapy. *Lancet Oncol* 2011; 12: 211–14.

2 Loehrer PJ Sr, Einhorn LH, Elson PJ, *et al.* A randomized comparison of cisplatin alone or in combination with methotrexate, vinblastine, and doxorubicin in patients with metastatic urothelial carcinoma: a cooperative group study. *J Clin Oncol* 1992; 10: 1066–73.

3 Logothetis CJ, Dexeus FH, Finn L, *et al.* A prospective randomized trial comparing MVAC and CISCA chemotherapy for patients with metastatic urothelial tumors. *J Clin Oncol* 1990; 8: 1050–5.

4 von der Maase H, Sengelov L, Roberts JT, *et al.* Long-term survival results of a randomized trial comparing gemcitabine plus cisplatin, with methotrexate, vinblastine, doxorubicin, plus cisplatin in patients with bladder cancer. *J Clin Oncol* 2005; 23: 4602–8.

5 Santis MD, Bellmunt J, Mead G, *et al.* Randomized phase II/III trial assessing gemcitabine/carboplatin and methotrexate/carboplatin/vinblastine in patients with advanced urothelial cancer who are unfit for cisplatin-based chemotherapy: EORTC study 30986. *J Clin Oncol* 2012; 30: 191–9.

6 Sharma P, Callahan MK, Bono P, *et al.* Nivolumab monotherapy in recurrent metastatic urothelial carcinoma (CheckMate 032): a multicentre, open-label, two-stage, multi-arm, phase 1/2 trial. *Lancet Oncol* 2016; 17: 1590–8.

7 Sharma P, Retz M, Siefker-Radtke A, *et al.* Nivolumab in metastatic urothelial carcinoma after platinum therapy (CheckMate 275): a multicentre, single-arm, phase 2 trial. *Lancet Oncol* 2017; 18: 312–22.

8 Bellmunt J, de Wit R, Vaughn DJ, *et al.* Pembrolizumab as second-line therapy for advanced urothelial carcinoma. *N Engl J Med* 2017; 376: 1015–26.

9 Powles T, Durán I, van der Heijden MS, *et al.* Atezolizumab versus chemotherapy in patients with platinum-treated locally advanced or metastatic urothelial carcinoma (IMvigor211): a multicentre, open-label, phase 3 randomised controlled trial. *Lancet* 2018; 391: 748–57.

10 Patel MR, Ellerton J, Infante JR, *et al.* Avelumab in metastatic urothelial carcinoma after platinum failure (JAVELIN Solid Tumor): pooled results from two expansion cohorts of an open-label, phase 1 trial. *Lancet Oncol* 2018; 19: 51–64.

11 Powles T, O'Donnell PH, Massard C, *et al*. Efficacy and safety of durvalumab in locally advanced or metastatic urothelial carcinoma: updated results from a phase 1/2 open-label study. *JAMA Oncol* 2017; 3: e172411.

12 Spain L, Diem S, Larkin J. Management of toxicities of immune checkpoint inhibitors. *Cancer Treat Rev* 2016; 44: 51–60.

13 Horvat TZ, Adel NG, Dang TO, *et al*. Immune-related adverse events, need for systemic immunosuppression, and effects on survival and time to treatment failure in patients with melanoma treated with ipilimumab at Memorial Sloan Kettering Cancer Center. *J Clin Oncol* 2015; 33: 3193–8.

Further reading

• Champiat S, Lambotte O, Barreau E, *et al*. Management of immune checkpoint blockade dysimmune toxicities: a collaborative position paper. *Ann Oncol* 2016; 27: 559–74.

• Medscape. *Sarcoidosis: practice essentials, background, pathophysiology*. Available from: https://emedicine.medscape.com/article/301914-overview (accessed 28 February 2018).

• Naidoo J, Page DB, Li BT, *et al*. Toxicities of the anti-PD-1 and anti-PD-L1 immune checkpoint antibodies. *Ann Oncol* 2015; 26: 2375–91.

• Suozzi KC, Stahl M, Ko CJ, *et al*. Immune-related sarcoidosis observed in combination ipilimumab and nivolumab therapy. *JAAD Case Rep* 2016; 2: 264–8.

20 Renal Cell Carcinoma Treated with Ipilimumab and Nivolumab

Maria Martinez, Balaji Venugopal

Case history

A 57-year-old man presented with haematuria and was diagnosed with locally advanced clear cell renal cell carcinoma (RCC) of the right kidney. He underwent radical nephrectomy, but 6 months later a surveillance CT scan of thorax, abdomen and pelvis revealed enlarged aortocaval lymph node and lung metastases. Multidisciplinary team review confirmed inoperable metastatic RCC. He was asymptomatic and had a WHO performance status score of 0 and no comorbidities. He was offered systemic anticancer therapy in a randomized phase III trial comparing the combination of ipilimumab plus nivolumab with sunitinib in advanced, untreated RCC. He was randomized to receive ipilimumab 1 mg/kg plus nivolumab 3 mg/kg intravenously every 3 weeks for four doses (induction phase), followed by nivolumab 3 mg/kg every 2 weeks (maintenance phase). He tolerated the first three doses of ipilimumab/nivolumab well but was admitted to hospital with abdominal pain, lethargy and headache 2 days prior to the fourth dose. Clinical examination of organ systems was normal and his haemodynamic parameters were stable.

He had deranged liver functions tests: alanine aminotransferase 7.41 µkat/l (range 0.17–0.68 µkat/l), aspartate aminotransferase 5.26 µkat/l (range 0.17–0.51 µkat/l), alkaline phosphatase 4.66 µkat/l (range 0.5–2.0 µkat/l), normal bilirubin, thyroid stimulating hormone 0.15 mIU/l (range 0.35–5.0 mIU/l), free thyroxine 5.1 pmol/l (range 9–21 pmol/l) and testosterone 4.8 nmol/l (range 10–36 nmol/l). Liver screen including coagulation, ultrasound, anti-nuclear antibodies, viral serology for hepatitis, immunoglobulins, caeruloplasmin, alpha-fetoprotein and coeliac serology was normal. MRI of brain and pituitary ruled out intracranial metastases or pituitary abnormalities.

The patient was diagnosed with immune checkpoint inhibitor (ICPI)-related hepatotoxicity and pituitary dysfunction. Treatment with corticosteroids normalized his liver function tests, but he required long-term replacement of thyroxine and testosterone.

What is the role of ICPIs in metastatic RCC?

What is the optimal dose of ipilimumab in combination with nivolumab?

What is the underlying mechanism of immune-related adverse events (irAEs)?

What is the clinical presentation and management of immune-related hepatitis?

What is the clinical presentation and management of immune-related endocrinopathies?

How should the patient's irAEs be managed?

What is the role of ICPIs in metastatic RCC?

RCC is an immunologically sensitive tumour. Older immunotherapy drugs such as interferon and high-dose interleukin produce a durable clinical response in some patients. The current era of immune checkpoint targeting of cytotoxic T lymphocyte-associated protein 4 (CTLA-4) and programmed cell death protein 1 (PD-1) or its ligand, programmed death-ligand 1 (PD-L1), has expanded the therapeutic options for inoperable and metastatic RCC.

On the basis of the results of the CheckMate 025 trial,[1] nivolumab, a monoclonal antibody against PD-1, was approved by the US Food and Drug Administration in individuals with RCC who had undergone prior treatment. CheckMate 025 demonstrated a 5 month improvement in overall survival (OS) in patients treated with nivolumab 3 mg/kg compared with everolimus (25.0 vs 19.6 months; HR for death 0.73; 98.5% CI 0.57, 0.93; $p=0.002$). The objective response rate was also greater with nivolumab compared with everolimus (25% vs 5%; odds ratio 5.98; 95% CI 3.68, 9.72; $p<0.001$).

More recently, the CheckMate 214 trial randomly assigned 1096 patients with intermediate and poor-risk previously untreated RCC to receive either nivolumab 3 mg/kg plus ipilimumab 1 mg/kg intravenously every 3 weeks for four doses, followed by nivolumab 3 mg/kg every 2 weeks, or sunitinib 50 mg orally once daily for 4 weeks (6 week cycle).[2] Response rates were improved in the immunotherapy group compared with the sunitinib group (42% vs 27%; $p<0.001$); 9% of patients in the immunotherapy group experienced a complete response vs 1% in the sunitinib group. The 18 month OS rate was 75% with nivolumab plus ipilimumab and 60% with sunitinib. The median OS was not reached in the nivolumab plus ipilimumab group and was 26.0 months in the sunitinib group (HR for death 0.63; $p<0.001$). Importantly, treatment-related adverse events occurred less frequently in the immunotherapy group compared with the sunitinib group, with grades 3–4 events occurring in 46% and 63% of patients, respectively.

Several ongoing clinical trials are evaluating the role of immunotherapeutic agents including ipilimumab (ClinicalTrials.gov NCT02231749), atezolizumab (ClinicalTrials.gov NCT02420821), avelumab (ClinicalTrials.gov NCT02684006) and pembrolizumab (ClinicalTrials.gov NCT02014636) as treatment for RCC in the adjuvant and metastatic settings.

What is the optimal dose of ipilimumab in combination with nivolumab?

Different doses and schedules of nivolumab plus ipilimumab have been chosen for investigation in different tumour types. For melanoma, nivolumab 1 mg/kg plus ipilimumab 3 mg/kg every 3 weeks for four cycles followed by nivolumab 240 mg every 2 weeks is the approved regimen. This was based on initial studies of single-agent ipilimumab at a dose of 3 mg/kg in initial early phase trials of ipilimumab and success at this dose observed in phase III studies.[3] For RCC, the regimen of nivolumab 3 mg/kg plus ipilimumab 1 mg/kg every 3 weeks for four cycles followed by nivolumab 3 mg/kg every 2 weeks seems to be optimal.[4] Differing doses and schedules of ipilimumab and nivolumab have been explored in a number of tumour types, most notably small-cell and non-small-cell lung carcinoma (NSCLC), in an attempt to ensure the best clinical outcome while reducing the risks of autoimmune side effects.[5,6] Combinations of nivolumab with low-dose ipilimumab ('ipi-lite') regimens appear to have good efficacy in RCC and NSCLC (ClinicalTrials.gov NCT01454102), and its benefit in melanoma and other tumours is currently being explored in clinical trials (ClinicalTrials.gov NCT03528408 and NCT03333616). It is interesting to note that the incidence of grades 3–4 toxicities with ipilimumab 3 mg/kg regimens is higher than with ipilimumab 1 mg/kg regimens. This low-dose ipilimumab combination was better tolerated than sunitinib in patients with RCC in the previously discussed phase III study.[2]

Reasons for tumour type-specific differences in tolerability and activity based on the dose and schedule of nivolumab and ipilimumab are unclear and require further study. It is uncertain whether differing doses are required according to tumour histology and site specificity. Interestingly, biomarker-specific approaches may also help determine which tumours are most likely to benefit from combination immunotherapy. Patients with NSCLC harbouring high mutational burdens respond better to combination immunotherapy than to cytotoxic chemotherapy.[7] The ultimate aim is to determine the optimal regimen for different tumour types that results in high responses and long-term OS gains and reduced toxicities.

What is the underlying mechanism of irAEs?

The exact pathophysiology of irAEs is not well defined. The therapeutic benefit of ICPIs is achieved by blocking immune inhibitory signals; the same mechanism results in acute and/or chronic activation of immune response and associated inflammation. T cell activation, antibodies and cytokines all play a role in irAEs. Whereas CTLA-4 attenuates the T cell response at the initiation phase, PD-1 inhibits the immune response in later stages in peripheral tissues, which explains the difference in the incidence of irAEs in CTLA-4 antibody and anti-PD-1/anti-PD-L1 antibodies. irAEs usually present a few weeks to a few months after initiating immunotherapy, but they may occur at any time point, even several months after discontinuation of immunotherapy. Clinicians must be vigilant about the possibility of irAEs in any patient who has had ICPI treatment. The severity of irAEs is graded according to the Common Terminology Criteria for Adverse Events.[8] In the absence of randomized trials, various guidelines and an expert consensus statement have been published and readers are advised to refer to these publications.[9-11]

What is the clinical presentation and management of immune-related hepatitis?

Immune-related hepatitis occurs in 5–10% of patients (1–2% grade 3) treated with ipilimumab, nivolumab or pembrolizumab monotherapy, and in 25–30% of patients (15% grade 3) treated with ipilimumab plus nivolumab.[2,3] Pooled analysis indicates a median time of onset and resolution of any grade hepatitis of 7.7 weeks (range 2.0–38.9 weeks) and 3.1 weeks (range 0.7–17.1 weeks), respectively, with nivolumab monotherapy, and a median time of onset and resolution of 6.1 weeks (range 0.1–49.7 weeks) and 4.6 weeks (range 0.1 to ≥53.1), respectively, for patients on ipilimumab/nivolumab combination therapy.[10,11] Immune-related hepatitis is mostly asymptomatic, but symptoms may include jaundice, abdominal pain, bruising, fatigue or fever. Patients should have liver function tests prior to each treatment and be assessed for signs and symptoms of hepatitis. Disease-related causes, biliary obstruction or thrombosis, concomitant drugs including alcohol intake, and infectious causes (viral hepatitis) should be ruled out. Immunosuppression with corticosteroids is the mainstay of treatment, together with prompt identification of irAEs and timely initiation of immunosuppressive and/or immunomodulatory agents.

What is the clinical presentation and management of immune-related endocrinopathies?

ICPI-related endocrine toxicities range from asymptomatic changes in thyroid function tests to adrenal crisis. Toxicities include thyroid dysfunction, hypophysitis, type 1 diabetes mellitus, adrenalitis, hypogonadism and hypoparathyroidism. Of these, thyroid dysfunction and hypophysitis are the commonest. Patients may present with fatigue, nausea and vomiting, headache, visual disturbances, diarrhoea, cold intolerance, hair loss, alteration in weight (gain or loss), hoarseness of voice, tachycardia, tremors, hypotension, hypoglycaemia and electrolyte imbalance. The median time to onset of any grade endocrinopathy with nivolumab monotherapy and ipilimumab/nivolumab combination therapy is 10.4 weeks (range 3.6–46.9 weeks) and 7.4 weeks (range 0.1–46.1 weeks), with median times to resolution of 28 weeks (range 0.9 to ≥48.1 weeks) and 42.7 weeks (range 0.4 to ≥93.9 weeks), respectively.[10,11]

Careful assessment of the patient's clinical history, to evaluate any underlying endocrine abnormality, and measurement of baseline thyroid function and glucose are indicated. The monitoring schedule varies according the type of ICPI; thyroid function may be checked every 3–4 weeks for the first 3 months and every 6–8 weeks subsequently.

How should the patient's irAEs be managed?

The patient suffered grade 3 hepatitis and was commenced on methylprednisolone 2 mg/kg daily. This produced a significant improvement in liver function within 3 days, after which he was switched to oral prednisolone at an equivalent dosage. His liver function returned to baseline and prednisolone was tapered over 4 weeks. He had persistent hypothyroidism and hypogonadism, however, which required long-term thyroxine and testosterone replacement. In view of his grade 3 hepatitis the ICPI was permanently discontinued and he was treated with anti-angiogenic agents as second line treatment for RCC.

Conclusion and learning points

- ICPIs have redefined the standard of care of different malignancies including RCC by achieving durable clinical responses and improving OS.
- ICPIs are generally well tolerated but they have a distinct toxicity profile; irAEs may happen at any time and even after termination of treatment and may be severe or fatal without prompt management.
- Educating patients and carers prior to initiation of treatment and during and following completion of treatment about the benefits, risks and long-term complications of ICPI is vital.
- The optimal dose of nivolumab and ipilimumab remains unclear and may differ depending on tumour type.

References

1 Motzer R, Escudier B, McDermott D, *et al*. Nivolumab versus everolimus in advanced renal cell carcinoma. *N Engl J Med* 2015; 373: 1803–13.

2 Motzer RJ, Tannir NM, McDermott DF, *et al*. Nivolumab plus ipilimumab versus sunitinib in advanced renal-cell carcinoma. *N Engl J Med* 2018; 378: 1277–90.

3 Larkin J, Chiaron S, González R, *et al*. Combined nivolumab and ipilimumab monotherapy in untreated melanoma. *N Engl J Med* 2015; 373: 23–34.

4 Hammers H, Plimack ER, Infante JR, *et al*. Expanded cohort results from CheckMate 016: a phase I study of nivolumab in combination with ipilimumab in metastatic renal cell carcinoma (mRCC). *J Clin Oncol* 2015; 33 (suppl): abstract 4516.

5 Antonia SJ, López-Martin JA, Bendell J, *et al*. Nivolumab alone and nivolumab plus ipilimumab in recurrent small-cell lung cancer (CheckMate 032): a multicentre, open-label, phase 1/2 trial. *Lancet Oncol* 2016; 17: 883–95.

6 Hellmann MD, Rizvi NA, Goldman JW, *et al*. Nivolumab plus ipilimumab as first-line treatment for advanced non-small-cell lung cancer (CheckMate 012): results of an open-label, phase 1, multicohort study. *Lancet Oncol* 2017; 18: 31–41.

7 Hellmann MD, Ciuleanu TE, Pluzansk A, *et al*. Nivolumab plus ipilimumab in lung cancer with a high tumor mutational burden. *N Engl J Med* 2018; 378: 2093–104.

8 US Department of Health and Human Services, National Institutes of Health, National Cancer Institute (2010). *Common Terminology Criteria for Adverse Events (CTCAE) v4.0*. Available from: https://ctep.cancer.gov/protocolDevelopment/electronic_applications/ctc. htm (accessed 14 August 2018).

9 Haanen JBAG, Carbonnel F, Robert C, *et al*. Management of toxicities from immunotherapy: ESMO clinical practice guidelines for diagnosis, treatment and follow-up. *Ann Oncol* 2017; 28 (suppl 4): iv119–42.

10 Brahmer JR, Lacchetti C, Schneider BJ, *et al*. Management of immune-related adverse events in patients treated with immune checkpoint inhibitor therapy: American Society of Clinical Oncology clinical practice guideline. *J Clin Oncol* 2018; 36: 1714–68.

11 Puzanov I, Diab A, Abdallah K, *et al*. Managing toxicities associated with immune checkpoint inhibitors: consensus recommendations from the Society for Immunotherapy of Cancer (SITC) Toxicity Management Working Group. *J Immunother Cancer* 2017; 5: 95.

21 Ocular Toxicity from Nivolumab

Andrew Viggars, Satinder Jagdev, Christy Ralph, Rosalind Stewart

Case history

 A 59-year-old woman with renal cell carcinoma (RCC) presented to the medical oncology clinic. Three years previously she had undergone a radical nephrectomy for a T3N0M0 clear cell carcinoma. She had no history of autoimmune disease and had previously been otherwise fit.

She was initially treated with interleukin (IL)-2 therapy, but it was complicated by a C2 vertebral fracture, after which she proceeded to further treatment with sunitinib. An initially good partial response was maintained for 30 months despite two dose reductions due to toxicities. Restaging scans at 30 months found further disease progression and she commenced nivolumab therapy.

After two cycles of nivolumab the patient presented with sore, red, dry eyes (more so in the left, where her vision had reduced to 6/24 unaided, 6/12 pinhole) and polyarthropathy involving the small joints of the hands and wrists. Both eyes were erythematous on examination. An urgent ophthalmology review noted blepharitis, bilateral conjunctival injection, and a marked left corneal epitheliopathy consistent with acute dry eye. She was prescribed hourly preservative-free topical lubricants and a lubricating ointment for night-time.

Three weeks later her symptoms had not improved. Her vision had deteriorated to 6/36 unaided, 6/18 pinhole in the left eye, and an inferior corneal infiltrate was noted typical of marginal keratitis. A punctual plug was inserted into the left lower punctum; she was commenced on topical levofloxacin six times a day and topical steroids were added 4 days later. Two weeks later, oral prednisolone 30 mg/day was commenced for ongoing symptoms. The polyarthropathy improved rapidly and her ocular symptoms gradually resolved. The dose of oral prednisolone was steadily reduced over 6 weeks.

Re-challenge with nivolumab was discussed, but it was not possible as her performance status declined prior to recommencing treatment.

What is the evidence for nivolumab treatment in RCC?

What are the differential diagnoses in this case?

Which ocular and orbital toxicities may patients experience with immunotherapy treatments?

How are ocular toxicities graded?

What is the management of ocular and orbital toxicity with immunotherapy?

What is the evidence for nivolumab treatment in RCC?

Nivolumab is a fully humanized immunoglobulin G4 antibody against programmed death-ligand 1 (PD-L1). It is licensed in the UK for the management of metastatic disease in RCC and in multiple other cancer tumour sites, and the list continues to grow as further trials show positive data. Recent data of combination immune checkpoint therapy (ipilimumab and nivolumab) show benefit in first line treatment and may lead to a change in practice.[1]

The CheckMate 025 trial reported in 2015 was a multicentre, multinational phase II trial comparing nivolumab with everolimus as second line treatment. It demonstrated a median overall survival (OS) advantage of 25.0 months for nivolumab vs 19.6 months for everolimus (HR 0.73). Partial responses were seen in 24% of patients on nivolumab compared with 5% in those receiving everolimus, and a favourable toxicity profile: grades 3–4 toxicities were seen in 19% of nivolumab-treated patients compared with 37% of everolimus-treated patients; the response was not dependent on PD-L1 expression. This trial did not include patients with non-clear cell carcinoma and required previous treatment with antiangiogenic therapies.[2]

In a phase II dose–response study in metastatic RCC patients pretreated with vascular endothelial growth factor (VEGF), tyrosine kinase inhibitors (TKIs) or monoclonal antibodies, overall response rates of 20–22% were seen.[3] Comparing dose responses demonstrated progression-free survival of 4.0 and 4.2 months in the 2 mg/kg and 10 mg/kg groups, respectively, with median OS of around 25 months. These results demonstrated that there is no dose-dependent response to nivolumab; therefore, lower doses may be used to achieve the same outcome with a lower risk of toxicity.

In 2016, NICE approved nivolumab for management of previously treated RCC. The recommendations were for use either as a second or third line agent after initial TKI treatment depending on comorbidities and the treating physician's choice.[4]

What are the differential diagnoses in this case?

Bilateral dry eyes and polyarthropathy raise the possibility of an autoimmune condition such as rheumatoid arthritis. Uveitis may also classically present alongside other autoimmune disorders, for example ankylosing spondylitis and inflammatory bowel disease. It is important to check for any concerning symptoms on systems enquiry.

Other causes of painful red eyes may include conjunctivitis, allergic eye disease, scleritis, uveitis, and emergencies such as angle closure glaucoma. An urgent ophthalmology review is thus imperative. Conjunctivitis and uveitis may be associated with reactive arthritis (though there were no urinary symptoms in this case).

Which ocular and orbital toxicities may patients experience with immunotherapy treatments?

Ocular toxicities from immunotherapy are rare, being reported in <1% of cases.[5] A range of ocular and orbital toxicities have been observed with immunotherapies, presenting at 1–12 weeks (median 2 months) after the start of treatment.[5] These include ocular inflammation, orbital inflammation and retinal/choroidal disease. The most serious ocular toxicity reported was loss of vision. Predominantly the literature reports toxicity after ipilimumab, which was the first licensed immune checkpoint inhibitor.

The most common event reported to date is uveitis, but a whole range of inflammatory eye conditions are recognized including episcleritis, conjunctivitis, blepharitis and dry eye (which are included on the summary of product characteristics for nivolumab as uncommon adverse events). Orbital toxicities include case reports describing Graves-like ophthalmopathy, ocular myasthenia and optic neuritis as complications of treatment. Retinal/choroidal disease includes choroidal neovascularization and melanoma-associated retinopathy. Vogt–Koyanagi–Harada disease (uveomeningoencephalitis, tinnitus or hearing loss, vitiligo and cranial nerve palsies) has been reported in patients on ipilimumab and pembrolizumab. Cataract has also been reported.[6]

These toxicities may occur in isolation, but combinations of the above are also reported. All of the above toxicities are uncommon but should prompt early ophthalmological assessment and consideration of temporary or permanent cessation of immunotherapy. All have the potential to cause significant morbidity and are potentially sight-threatening. As with other toxicities of treatment, the risk of ocular toxicity increases with combination immunotherapy (for example, ipilimumab and nivolumab).

How are ocular toxicities graded?

Ocular and orbital toxicities can be graded according to the Common Terminology Criteria for Adverse Events (CTCAE). There are multiple different types of ophthalmic disorders that may be graded; however, in terms of those relating to immunotherapy, most follow the same pattern:

- grade 1: asymptomatic with clinical or diagnostic observations only;

- grade 2: symptomatic, requiring medical intervention and limiting instrumental activities of daily living;

- grade 3: symptomatic, affecting visual acuity (worse than 6/120) and limiting self-care activities of daily living;

- grade 4: blindness (6/60 or worse) in the affected eye.

The diagnosis of eye/orbital disease requires assessment by an ophthalmologist, using methods including visual field assessment and slit lamp investigation and investigations such as retinal optical coherence tomography. Of note, colitis and eye toxicity may coexist; therefore, in patients presenting with colitis, a history should be taken to exclude eye disease.

Grading is usually used to help guide the therapeutic options and further management of the patient. No such treatment algorithms are, however, available for ocular and orbital toxicity. Nevertheless, grading does allow correct documentation of severity at diagnosis (baseline), response to treatment and inter-specialty communication of severity.

What is the management of ocular and orbital toxicity with immunotherapy?

There is as yet no defined treatment algorithm for the management of ocular toxicity, owing to a paucity of data. Similar to other immunotherapy-related toxicities, grade 1 toxicities may be managed expectantly with continuation of treatment and close observation over subsequent cycles of treatment. In any toxicity greater than grade 1, treatment should be suspended, and an ophthalmic review should be sought to ensure a correct diagnosis is made and management plan instigated. It may also be necessary to seek a neurological review if there is concern about optic nerve involvement or myasthenic symptoms.

Management of ocular and orbital toxicities will vary greatly depending on the specific diagnosis and should be guided by the treating ophthalmologist. Steroids for inflammatory conditions may be administered topically or by periocular injection, although systemic treatment is usually required for severe disease.

With eye disorders and immunotherapy there is the potential for topical, rather than systemic, therapy in the initial management (grade 2 or less). Topical ciclosporin has been reported with good effect in two cases of dry eye associated with nivolumab.[7] As with all cases of toxicity from immunotherapy in one organ system, it is also prudent to ensure that screening is carried out for other organ system dysfunction. Screening should include a full history and examination, and basic investigations such as a full blood count, liver function tests, hormone profiles, fasting glucose measurement, basic biochemistry and urine dipstick to ensure no other toxicities are present.[8] Further investigations should be guided by clinical findings.

Conclusion

- Ocular and orbital toxicities from immunotherapy, although uncommon, are wide ranging and may be part of multisystem disorders.
- Screening (history and clinical examination) should be considered in all patients presenting with immune colitis, because of its reported coexistence.
- Grading is assessed by specific CTCAE guidance to aid inter-specialty communication and accurate documentation.
- Early involvement of ophthalmologists is required for all toxicities higher than grade 1.
- Recovery may be relatively swift with early management; toxicity can sometimes be controlled with topical agents only.

References

1 Motzer R, Tannir N, McDermott D, *et al*. Nivolumab plus ipilimumab versus sunitinib in advanced renal-cell carcinoma. *N Engl J Med* 2018; 378: 1277–90.

2 Motzer R, Rini B, McDermott D, *et al*. Nivolumab for metastatic renal cell carcinoma: results of a randomized phase II trial. *J Clin Oncol* 2015; 33: 1430–7.

3 Motzer R, Escudier B, McDermott D, *et al*. Nivolumab versus everolimus for advanced renal cell carcinoma. *N Engl J Med* 2015; 373: 1803–13.

4 National institute for Health and Care Excellence (2016). *Nivolumab for previously treated advanced renal cell carcinoma. Technology appraisal guidance TA417*. Available from: www.nice.org.uk/guidance/ta417 (accessed 18 February 2018).

5 Antouna J, Titah C, Cochereau I. Ocular and orbital side-effects of checkpoint inhibitors: a review article. *Curr Opin Oncol* 2016; 28: 288–94.

6 Abdel-Rahman O, Oweira H, Petrausch U, *et al*. Immune-related ocular toxicities in solid tumor patients treated with immune checkpoint inhibitors: a systematic review. *Exp Rev Anticancer Ther* 2017; 17: 387–94.

7 Nguyen AT, Elia M, Materin MA, *et al*. Cyclosporine for dry eye associated with nivolumab. A case progressing to corneal perforation. *Cornea* 2016; 35: 399–401.

8 Haanen JBAG, Carbonnel F, Robert C, *et al*. Management of toxicities from immunotherapy: ESMO clinical practice guidelines for diagnosis, treatment and follow-up. *Ann Oncol* 2017; 28 (suppl 4): iv119–42.

22 Multiple Immune-Related Toxicities in a Patient with Breast Cancer on Immune Checkpoint Inhibition and Chemotherapy

Rachel Broadbent, Andrew M. Wardley

Case history

A 49-year-old woman presented with a 6 cm left breast mass and was diagnosed with invasive ductal carcinoma, oestrogen receptor (ER) 0, progesterone receptor (PR) 0, human epidermal growth factor receptor 2 (HER2) 0, and a left axillary node and liver metastases. She had no medical history and her performance status was 0. She took no medications.

She was enrolled on phase III of the IMpassion130 trial in which patients with previously untreated metastatic triple-negative breast cancer were randomised either to atezolizumab (840 mg) 2 weekly plus nab-paclitaxel (100 mg/m²) 3 weeks on/1 week off or to placebo 2 weekly plus nab-paclitaxel (100 mg/m²) 3 weeks on/1 week off.

At cycle 3 she developed a grade 3 rise in aspartate aminotransferase (AST), which was treated with a single dose of methylprednisolone 1 mg/kg followed by 60 mg prednisolone/day. Nab-paclitaxel plus atezolizumab or placebo were withheld for 2 and 4 weeks, respectively. Prednisolone was weaned over 8 weeks and there were no further AST rises.

At cycle 7, amylase was checked as part of a routine blood test and found to be 5.95 μkat/l (grade 3 rise). The patient was asymptomatic. All trial treatment was withheld. An abdominal ultrasound revealed an unremarkable pancreas and no mass. Magnetic resonance cholangiopancreatography (MRCP) showed no evidence of pancreatitis or collection. After 42 days the patient restarted trial treatment following discussion with the medical monitor. The trends in amylase and liver enzymes are shown in Table 22.1 (not all results are consecutive).

At cycle 11 the patient reported grade 1 diarrhoea, which was controlled with loperamide. She continued on trial treatment. The results of investigations at this time are shown in Table 22.2. A planned CT scan 8 weeks later showed mural thickening of the sigmoid colon; therefore, treatment was withheld. At this time, diarrhoea was grades 1–2. A colonoscopy and biopsy revealed colitis and proctitis up to the descending colon. Prednisolone was commenced (40 mg/day).

Nab-paclitaxel and placebo or atezolizumab were restarted after 4 and 6 weeks, respectively, when symptoms were resolved. At this time the patient remained on prednisolone 20 mg/day. Attempts to wean prednisolone further over the next 10 months resulted in recurrent grades 1–2 diarrhoea requiring further steroids. Oral sulfasalazine was trialled but discontinued due to nausea.

A CT scan at cycle 22 showed worsening inflammation of the rectum and sigmoid colon with appearance of ulceration but otherwise stable disease. The prednisolone dose was escalated to 80 mg/day. Nab-paclitaxel was continued; however, atezolizumab or placebo were withheld.

Table 22.1 Trend in liver enzyme abnormalities.

Time point (cycle C, day D)	AST, μkat/l (ref. range 0.17–0.51)	ALP, μkat/l (ref. range 0.5–2.0)	Bilirubin, μmol/l (ref. range 1–20)	GGT, μkat/l (ref. range 0.03–0.51)	Amylase, μkat/l (ref. range 0.46–2.23)
C3D1	2.49	2.3	7	1.32	NA
C3D8	6.06	2.54	6	1.55	NA
C3D11	2.20	2.27	6	1.64	NA
C3D15	1.12	1.90	6	1.57	NA
C7D1	0.52	1.84	6	0.72	4.29
C7D15	0.53	1.90	7	0.75	6.21
C7D29	0.42	1.89	6	0.68	4.24
C7D43	0.43	1.77	6	0.68	2.45

ALP, alkaline phosphatase; GGT, gamma glutamyltransferase.

Table 22.2 Investigations at onset of diarrhoea.

Investigation	Result
WBC, ×10^9/l	4.7
Neutrophil count, ×10^9/l	6.2
Creatinine, μmol/l	77
eGFR, ml min^{-1} (1.73 m)$^{-2}$	78
Bilirubin, μmol/l	7
ALP, μkat/l	1.52
AST, μkat/l	0.43
Free T$_4$, pmol/l (range)	12.3 (10–22)
TSH, mIU/l (range)	9.05 (0.55–4.78)
Stool culture	Reported negative by GP surgery

ALP, alkaline phosphatase; eGFR, estimated glomerular filtration rate; T$_4$, thyroxine; TSH, thyroid-stimulating hormone; WBC, white blood cell count.

In terms of tumour response, at baseline she had a 5.7 cm left breast mass, which was no longer measurable at the cycle 22 scan. At cycle 22 her liver metastases were stable. The left axillary nodes were seen to be increasing in size from cycle 6. A CT-guided biopsy of one of the axillary nodes was performed at cycle 12, which revealed granulomatous lymphadenitis with no malignancy. The lymph nodes began to reduce in size at cycle 19.

How should immunotherapy-related colitis be managed?

To what extent was the patient's colitis treated according to clinical guidance, and what evidence is available in the literature?

How common is immunotherapy-related hyperamylasaemia and pancreatitis, and how should they be managed?

How did the management of this patient's hyperamylasaemia affect the clinical outcome?

How should immunotherapy-related colitis be managed?

Colitis may be graded using the Common Terminology Criteria for Adverse Events (CTCAE) published by the National Cancer Institute.[1] Guidance on grading is also available in the European Society for Medical Oncology (ESMO) guidelines on management of immune toxicities.[2] Grading according to these guidelines is shown in Table 22.3.

According to the ESMO guidelines,[2] symptomatic management of diarrhoea of any grade should include loperamide, oral fluids and a low fibre diet. Investigations should include bloods (full blood count, urea and electrolytes, liver function test, thyroid function test, C-reactive protein) and stool microscopy for leucocytes/ova/parasites, culture, viral polymerase chain reaction, *Clostridium difficile* toxin and *Cryptosporidium*. Further investigations should include an abdominal film if the patient has pain, and a sigmoidoscopy/colonoscopy (± biopsy). The treatment options for immune-related colitis according to the ESMO guidelines[2] are summarized in Table 22.4.

Table 22.3 Grading of diarrhoea according to ESMO and CTCAE.

Grade	ESMO	CTCAE
1	Mild: <4 liquid stools/day over baseline; feeling well	Asymptomatic, clinical or diagnostic observations only; intervention not needed
2	Moderate: 4–6 liquid stools/day over baseline or abdominal pain; blood in stool; nausea or nocturnal episodes	Abdominal pain; mucus or blood in stool
3	Severe: >6 liquid stools/day over baseline or episodes within an hour of eating	Severe abdominal pain; change in bowel habits; medical intervention indicated; peritoneal signs
4		Life-threatening consequences; urgent intervention needed

Table 22.4 Management of immune-mediated colitis according to ESMO guidelines.

Event	Management
Grade 1 diarrhoea >14 days or grade 2 diarrhoea >3 days	Initiate baseline investigations and symptomatic management
	Commence prednisolone 0.5–1.0 mg/kg per day
Grade 3 or 4 diarrhoea OR Grade 1–2 diarrhoea not improved within 72 h	Commence methylprednisolone 1–2 mg/kg per day
If no improvement to grade 3 or 4 diarrhoea within 72 h	Infliximab 5 mg/kg stat
	Infliximab may be repeated after 2 weeks
	Mycophenolate mofetil 500–1000 mg twice daily and tacrolimus are other immunosuppressive treatment options

Oral steroids should be weaned over a period of 4–8 weeks depending on symptom severity. Immune checkpoint inhibitor (ICPI) treatment may continue if symptoms are grade 1, but should be withheld for grade 2. A dietary review and CT scan should be considered. Rectal bleeding and abdominal pain or distension should merit a surgical review. Contraindications to infliximab include hepatitis, TB, sepsis or New York Heart Association class III/IV heart failure.

To what extent was the patient's colitis treated according to clinical guidance, and what evidence is available in the literature?

When the patient first presented with grade 1 diarrhoea, appropriate investigations were performed (Table 22.2). The patient was found to be hypothyroid; therefore, levothyroxine was commenced. Loperamide was initiated and the trial treatment continued. Colonoscopy was performed around 7 weeks after the patient's grade 1 diarrhoea began. Guidance would suggest this should have been performed when symptoms had persisted for more than 7 days.[2]

A case series of patients on programmed cell death protein 1 (PD-1) or programmed death-ligand 1 (PD-L1) inhibitors who developed clinical features of colitis found that of 17 patients who underwent colonoscopy and biopsy, six had normal mucosa, three had mild colitis, and the remaining eight had marked changes including erosion and friability.[3] Of the six with normal mucosa, four had diarrhoea which resolved on discontinuation of the drug or on commencing immunosuppressive agents, suggesting it was related to the PD-1/PD-L1 inhibitor. These four patients had been on treatment for between 1 and 6 months and had had diarrhoea for between 3 days and 4 months. It could therefore be argued that colonoscopy is not sensitive for diagnosing immune-mediated colitis, and an earlier colonoscopy might not have changed the management and outcome. Conversely, if an earlier colonoscopy had been performed and shown colitis, steroid therapy might have been commenced earlier.

When grade 2 diarrhoea was recorded, atezolizumab or placebo were correctly withheld. Prednisolone was commenced at a dose of 0.5 mg/kg per day. According to guidance this should have been a dose of 1–2 mg/kg per day. Oral sulfasalazine was trialled with permission from the sponsor but discontinued. According to guidance a referral to a gastroenterologist should have been made.

The benefits of infliximab in treating acute severe ulcerative colitis in patients with corticosteroid-dependent colitis are well known. Infliximab reduces the incidence of colectomy in acute severe colitis and may induce clinical and endoscopic remission in corticosteroid-dependent colitis.[4] Currently the ESMO guidelines[2] advocate the use of infliximab in patients with steroid-resistant colitis with grades 3–4 diarrhoea, but do not discuss its potential use in corticosteroid-dependent colitis with a lower grade of symptomatology. This demonstrates the discrepancies between the well-established medical treatments for ulcerative colitis and the treatment of immunotherapy-related colitis and highlights the need for gastroenterology input.

There are few data regarding the safety of resuming anti-PD-1/anti-PD-L1 antibodies after immune-related adverse events (irAEs). In this case, atezolizumab or placebo was recommenced after 6 weeks, when diarrhoea was resolved, and the patient had weaned prednisolone to 20 mg/day. Following re-initiation, atezolizumab or placebo were continued, while the patient required prednisolone doses of up to 30 mg/day. The ESMO guidelines[2] recommend a slow weaning course of steroids over 6–8 weeks following colitis. While the guidelines do not specify a steroid dosage at which ICPI therapy may be resumed following colitis, in the case of pneumonitis it is recommended to be 10 mg/day.

A study of patients with metastatic melanoma who resumed anti-PD-1 therapy after discontinuation of combined anti-cytotoxic T lymphocyte-associated protein 4 (CTLA-4)/PD-1 blockade due to irAEs found that only 8% of patients who discontinued due to colitis had recurrent colitis on resumption of PD-1 blockade.[5] In patients with any previous irAEs who had a recurrent or distinct irAE, ongoing steroids at the time of resumption seemed to be a risk factor for a further irAE. It is not possible to tell based on such limited data whether this patient's clinical outcome would have been different had atezolizumab or placebo been withheld until steroids were discontinued.

A CT scan at cycle 22 showed worsening inflammation of the rectum and sigmoid colon with the appearance of ulceration. The patient was reporting grades 1–2 symptoms. This highlights the discrepancy between the severity of reported symptoms and imaging findings.

How common is immunotherapy-related hyperamylasaemia and pancreatitis, and how should they be managed?

In the Electronic Medicines Compendium summary of product characteristics for atezolizumab, pancreatitis is described as an uncommon, undesirable effect occurring in <1% of treated patients, while an amylase increase is a rare effect occurring in <0.1% of treated patients.[6] The ESMO guidelines describe pancreatitis as a possible side effect associated with CTLA-4-induced enterocolitis and a rare side effect of combined anti-CTLA-4 and anti-PD-1 antibodies.[2] It is recommended that when pancreatitis occurs, immunotherapy is discontinued and immunosuppression commenced. The guidelines do not describe treatment of raised amylase/lipase if the patient does not have a clinical diagnosis of pancreatitis.[2]

How did the management of this patient's hyperamylasaemia affect the clinical outcome?

The patient was asymptomatic throughout the episode of hyperamylasaemia. Atezolizumab or placebo were correctly withheld on discovery of the grade 3 event. Investigations including an abdominal ultrasound and MRCP did not identify a cause of the raised amylase. During this time the amylase levels were monitored weekly and showed spontaneous improvement to grade 1 within 7 weeks, so atezolizumab or placebo was appropriately restarted following discussion with the medical monitor.

Conclusion and learning points

- Multiple irAEs may occur in patients treated with anti-PD-1/anti-PD-L1 antibodies. There are currently no available biomarkers to predict which patients will develop these toxicities; therefore, clinicians must be vigilant and consent patients appropriately.

- Colitis may present with grades 1–2 diarrhoea; persistent symptoms may be debilitating and should be treated aggressively according to current ESMO guidelines.[2] Worsening of imaging appearances of colitis may not correlate with deteriorating symptoms.

- Clinicians should exercise caution when resuming/continuing anti-PD-1/anti-PD-L1 antibody treatment in patients who have had an irAE, especially when there is an ongoing steroid requirement. There is evidence to suggest that such patients may have recurrent or distinct irAEs on resumption of therapy.[6]

- Pancreatic events including hyperamylasaemia and pancreatitis are rare known side effects of anti-PD-1/anti-PD-L1 antibody treatment. Further research is required.

References

1   US Department of Health and Human Services (2017). *Common Terminology Criteria for Adverse Events, version 5.0*. Available from: https://ctep.cancer.gov/protocolDevelopment/electronic_applications/docs/CTCAE_v5_Quick_Reference_5x7.pdf (accessed 25 June 2018).

2   Haanen JBAG, Carbonnel F, Robert C, *et al*. Management of toxicities from immunotherapy: ESMO clinical practice guidelines for diagnosis, treatment and follow-up. *Ann Oncol* 2017; 28 (suppl 4): iv119–42.

3   González RS, Salaria SN, Bohannon CD *et al*. PD-1 inhibitor gastroenterocolitis: case series and appraisal of 'immunomodulatory gastroenterocolitis'. *Histopathology* 2017; 70: 558–67.

4   Burger D, Travis S. Conventional medical management of inflammatory bowel disease. *Gastroenterology* 2011; 140: 1827–37.

5   Pollack MH, Betof A, Dearden H, *et al*. Safety of resuming anti-PD-1 in patients with immune-related adverse events during combined anti-CTLA-4 and anti-PD1 in metastatic melanoma. *Ann Oncol* 2018; 29: 250–5.

6   eMC (2018). *Tecentriq 1,200 mg concentrate for solution for infusion*. Available from: www.medicines.org.uk/emc/product/8442/smpc (accessed 11 May 2018).

Further reading

- De Valasco G, Je Y, Bosse D, *et al*. Comprehensive meta-analysis of key immune-related adverse events from CTLA-4 and PD-1/PD-L1 inhibitors in cancer patients. *Cancer Immunol Res* 2017; 5: 312–18.

- Schmid P, Cruz C, Braiteh FE, *et al*. Atezolizumab in metastatic TNBC: long-term clinical outcomes and biomarker analysis. Presented at: American Association for Cancer Research annual meeting, 3 April 2017. Abstract 2986.

CASE STUDY

23 Oncolytic Viral Therapy: Talimogene Laherparepvec

Maria Marples

Case history

A 68-year-old woman had her left great toe amputated for a 3.8 mm Breslow thickness ulcerated acral lentiginous subungual melanoma with microsatellites. Sentinel node biopsy showed multiple parenchymal deposits of melanoma; subsequent inguinal node dissection showed melanoma deposits in three of eight nodes. A staging CT scan was clear. *BRAF* mutation status was wild-type.

Two years after initial surgery she developed in-transit metastases in the left leg, treated with excision and cryoablation. She then presented in the plastic surgery clinic with painful fungating nodules measuring up to 1 cm on the left leg, groin and buttock. Her performance status was 1.

Her medical history included hypertension (with a non-ST segment elevation myocardial infarction 3 months previously), rheumatoid arthritis and non-insulin-dependent diabetes mellitus. She was taking aspirin, ramipril, bendroflumethiazide, naproxen and metformin. A reassessment CT scan of the head, neck, chest, abdomen and pelvis showed no visceral metastases. Her lactate dehydrogenase (LDH) level was 3.01 µkat/l (normal range 1.7–3.4 µkat/l).

She was treated with talimogene laherparepvec (T-VEC). After two treatments she had fever of 38 °C, managed with paracetamol. She had paracetamol premedication with subsequent cycles and had no further fevers. During the first 3 months she developed new lesions but remained well, so treatment continued. At 6 months her disease was noted to be stable.

How did *BRAF* testing influence the treatment options for this patient?

What is T-VEC, and what is the evidence base for treating melanoma patients with it?

How is T-VEC administered?

How should treatment be modified in patients who develop new lesions while receiving T-VEC?

What extra precautions should patients take while they are being treated with T-VEC?

How did *BRAF* testing influence the treatment options for this patient?

In common with most acral lentiginous melanomas, the patient's tumour did not exhibit a mutation in the *BRAF* gene. Serine/threonine-protein kinase B-Raf (BRAF) inhibitor therapy was therefore not appropriate. Immunotherapy with checkpoint inhibitors was precluded by her rheumatoid arthritis. Cytotoxic chemotherapy with dacarbazine has a low objective response rate of 10–20% and does not prolong survival.

The patient had previously been treated with excisions and cryoablation of her lesions. As the lesions were now more extensive, electrochemotherapy could have been considered, but it was not appropriate as she would have needed a general anaesthetic, which is contraindicated in patients who have had a recent myocardial infarction. Radiotherapy could have been used for lesions that were painful or bleeding, but it would not have controlled all her disease.

T-VEC has a European licence for use in adults who have unresectable melanoma that is regionally or distantly metastatic (stages IIIB, IIIC and IVM1a) and no bone, brain, lung or other visceral deposits.[1] At least one lesion must be accessible for injection: cutaneous, subcutaneous and nodal metastases are acceptable. In addition, NICE guidance TA410 specifies that treatment with T-VEC may be considered if systemically administered immunotherapies are not suitable for the patient, and a discount agreed in the patient access scheme should be provided by the manufacturer.[2]

As this patient's disease could not be controlled by radiotherapy or surgery, and systemic therapies were unsuitable, treatment with T-VEC was recommended.

What is T-VEC, and what is the evidence base for treating melanoma patients with it?

T-VEC (previously known as OncoVEX[GM-CSF]) is a genetically engineered oncolytic herpes simplex virus type 1 (HSV-1).[3] Modifications include: deletion of the gene encoding infected cell protein (ICP) 34.5, leading to replication in cancer cells but not normal tissues; deletion of the gene encoding ICP 47, which enhances anti-tumour responses; and insertion of the human gene encoding granulocyte macrophage colony-stimulating factor (GM-CSF), which, when expressed, enhances the immune response when the cancer cell lyses and releases tumour antigens. T-VEC in melanoma patients has been tested in three studies.

- Phase I: the Biovex Study 001/01 was the first human study of T-VEC and included 30 patients with injectable lesions from various cancers, nine of whom had melanoma.[4] Some injected lesions were observed to flatten; regression of a lesion that had not been injected was also observed.

- Phase II: this trial was a single-arm study of T-VEC in 50 patients with injectable melanoma lesions.[5] Thirteen patients (26%) had an objective response to treatment, six of whom had initial progression with new lesions appearing. Around half of patients experienced flu-like symptoms, but grades 3–4 adverse events were rare.

- Phase III: the OPTiM trial was for patients with cutaneous metastatic melanoma with at least one injectable lesion >1 cm, good performance status, LDH <1.5 times the upper limit of normal, and limited visceral disease.[6] Patients (n=436) were randomized 2:1 to intralesional T-VEC or subcutaneous GM-CSF. The primary endpoint was durable response rate (the rate of objective response lasting for at least 6 months and beginning within 12 months of the start of treatment); secondary endpoints included overall survival (OS) and response rate. After a median follow-up of 44.4 months the durable response rate for T-VEC was 16.3% compared with 2.1% for GM-CSF; the difference was greatest in patients with unresectable stage III (33% vs 0%) or stage IV M1a (16% vs 2%) melanoma. The overall response rate was 26.4% for T-VEC and 5.7% for GM-CSF. Median OS was 23.3 months for T-VEC and 18.9 months for GM-CSF. Again, chills and fevers were common with T-VEC, as was injection-site pain (28% of patients).

How is T-VEC administered?

T-VEC is injected intralesionally. The maximum volume of the preparation is 4 ml, which is divided among the lesions to be injected. Priority is given to larger lesions and symptomatic lesions; as treatment continues, new lesions should be injected first. Not all lesions need to be injected. Ultrasound guidance may be needed for deeper lesions such as lymph nodes.[1]

Patients may be given premedication such as paracetamol 1 g. Local anaesthetic is not usually required, but if it is used it should be injected around (not into) the lesion. T-VEC is injected in a fan-like manner using a single entry point (Figures 23.1–23.3). A new needle should be used for each lesion. Injection sites should be covered with occlusive dressings that may be removed 1 week later.

The first T-VEC treatment is given at a lower concentration of T-VEC (10^6 plaque-forming units [PFU]/ml), which is designed to seroconvert patients who are HSV-negative. The next treatment is given 3 weeks later at full dose (10^8 PFU/ml) and continues 2 weekly.[1]

T-VEC is a live virus which is not expected to cause disease in healthy humans. Additional precautions, however, are generally taken when T-VEC is given. Staff should wear gloves, a gown or apron, and eye protection. Staff who are pregnant or immunocompromised should not handle T-VEC. Patients may be treated in a bay. Any spills should be cleaned up with a 1:10 solution of bleach in water using absorbent materials. Any materials that have been in contact with T-VEC should be placed in a plastic bag and disposed of in general waste.[1]

How should treatment be modified in patients who develop new lesions while receiving T-VEC?

Patients may develop new lesions while on T-VEC treatment. In the OPTiM trial, 42/78 of patients (54%) who had a response to T-VEC had initial progression.[6] The manufacturer's recommendation is therefore to continue treatment with T-VEC for at least 6 months unless there is

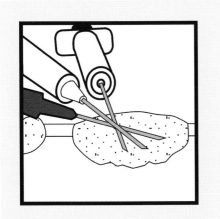

Figure 23.1 Injection administration for cutaneous lesions (adapted from Electronic Medicines Compendium[1] by D. Marples).

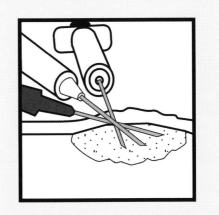

Figure 23.2 Injection administration for subcutaneous lesions (adapted from Electronic Medicines Compendium[1] by D. Marples).

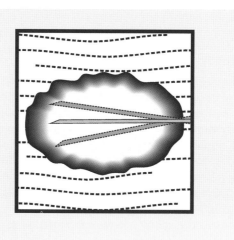

Figure 23.3 Injection administration for nodal lesions (adapted from Electronic Medicines Compendium[1] by D. Marples).

clinically significant progression or a drop in performance status requiring a change in therapy. If new lesions develop and are accessible, they should be injected first. If all lesions disappear and new ones appear later, they may also be treated with T-VEC.

What extra precautions should patients take while they are being treated with T-VEC?

Patients should keep their injection sites covered with occlusive dressings for 1 week, or longer if lesions are weeping. If a dressing comes off, it should be replaced. Dressings should be handled with gloves. Dressings, wipes, gloves and any other materials that might have been in contact with T-VEC should be placed in a plastic bag which should be tied shut and discarded in household waste.

Patients do not need to be isolated from other people. They should, however, avoid allowing their injection sites to come into contact with others, especially pregnant or immunocompromised people. Patients or their contacts who develop herpetic lesions should have polymerase chain reaction analysis for HSV typing and may be treated with aciclovir.

Conclusion and learning points

- T-VEC is a treatment option for patients with unresectable stages IIIB–IVM1a melanoma who have injectable lesions.
- Treatment with T-VEC is usually well tolerated; the main side effects are flu-like symptoms and pain at the injection site.
- Patients treated with T-VEC should usually continue treatment for at least 6 months if they are well enough, even if new lesions occur, as they may then develop a response.

References

1   Electronic Medicines Compendium (2018). *Imlygic summary of product characteristics.* Available from: www.medicines.org.uk/emc/product/5117 (accessed 25 March 2018).

2   National Institute for Health and Care Excellence (2016). *Talimogene laherparepvec for treating unresectable metastatic melanoma. Technology appraisal guidance TA410.* Available from: www.nice.org.uk/guidance/ta410 (accessed 25 March 2018).

3   Liu BL, Robinson M, Han ZQ, *et al.* ICP34.5 deleted herpes simplex virus with enhanced oncolytic, immune stimulating, and anti-tumour properties. *Gene Ther* 2003; 10: 292–303.

4   Hu JCC, Coffin RS, Davis CJ, *et al.* A phase I study of OncoVEX^GM-CSF, a second-generation oncolytic herpes simplex virus expressing granulocyte macrophage colony-stimulating factor. *Clin Cancer Res* 2006; 12: 6737–47.

5   Senzer NN, Kaufman HL, Amatruda T, *et al.* Phase II clinical trial of a granulocyte-macrophage colony-stimulating factor-encoding, second-generation oncolytic herpesvirus in patients with unresectable metastatic melanoma. *J Clin Oncol* 2009; 27: 5763–71.

6   Andtbacka RHI, Kaufman HL, Collichio F, *et al.* Talimogene laherparepvec improves durable response rate in patients with advanced melanoma. *J Clin Oncol* 2015; 33: 2780–8.

Further reading

•   Harrington KJ, Puzanov I, Hecht RJ, *et al.* Clinical development of talimogene laherparepvec (T-VEC): a modified herpes simplex virus type-1-derived oncolytic immunotherapy. *Exp Rev Anticancer Ther* 2015; 15: 1389–403.

•   Kaufman HL, Amatruda T, Reid T, *et al.* Systemic versus local responses in melanoma patients treated with talimogene laherparepvec from a multi-institutional phase II study. *J Immunother Cancer* 2016; 4: 12.

•   Seery V. Intralesional therapy. Consensus statements for best practices in administration from the Melanoma Nursing Initiative. *Clin J Oncol Nurs* 2017; 21 (4 suppl): 76–86.

Index